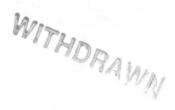

To the one who amazes me most,

my wonderful husband, Dan—

I made a wish and you came true.

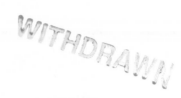

Contents

Foreword

Morbid obesity has become one of the most important health-care issues of our times. It is perhaps, in great part, a by-product of our success and affluence, but it could eventually contribute to our demise if not brought under control. The cost, in health-care dollars and in human suffering, is staggering and getting worse despite our best efforts.

Bariatric surgery plays a role in helping some of the millions of those afflicted with this disease and its terrible consequences, but it is not by any means the answer to the problem. We must gain control of this issue with education at the lowest levels. Teaching our children by example, beginning at home and in our schools, will, it is hoped, curb this trend.

What we have in this book is the story of two remarkable people who have made a dramatic change in their lives and who have become great advocates for a better way of life. Their enthusiasm and generosity have touched many lives for the better. Their dedication to helping others in this long process, which relies heavily on a strong support structure, has included patient-run support groups, Internet support sessions providing extensive information, and biweekly chat rooms. They also take time from their busy schedule to visit post-op patients and promote this practice to other post-op patients.

This book should serve as a guide to help those seeking this tool to become healthier and make those necessary changes to overcome their illness.

I have become a better person and doctor through their loving influence, and I am forever grateful to them for their friendship.

ALFREDO FERNANDEZ, M.D.
Director of Bariatrics, Brandon Regional Hospital,
Tampa, Florida

Acknowledgments

THE THANKS and acknowledgments are many and sincerely from the heart:

- Al Fernandez and Martha Rivera-Fernandez came into our lives, saved our lives, changed our lives, and are now part of our lives forever. Our love and admiration for them is for always.
- Mary Krupa set this whole book in motion without even realizing it. It was her urging from within our support family that set the foundation for this endeavor.
- Laura Nolan is the best literary agent anyone could ask to have. I've relied on you and counted on you, and I so appreciate you.
- Sarah Pelz, my publisher, has worked diligently, listened thoughtfully, and been encouraging at every turn.
- Elaine Poston has been the teacher who encouraged me and urged me on.

- For the members of our support family who shared their stories in this book, thank you for giving of yourselves so others can learn and be inspired by each of you.
- My parents, Nancy and Robert Gordon, love us unconditionally and endlessly.
- JT Parish, my brother-in-law, had the all-time best post-op experience.
- Virginia Thornton, my mother-in-law, has always been there with love and encouragement.
- Phyllis Schieber, my dear friend through so many years, your feedback, support, and friendship are priceless to me.
- To our support family, both local and online, without you, this book would not have been possible. You are the most genuine and loving support family anywhere.

Taking a Peek at Your Bright Future

SOMETHING AMAZING happened after my husband, Dan, and I had weight-loss surgery. The amazing thing wasn't that we had this procedure together, on the same day, in the same hospital, with the same surgeon. It wasn't just losing weight, even though in the following eight months, we had lost 300 pounds between us. It was a combination of everything. Triggered by the surgery, our health began improving from the very first day. The weight loss reversed medical conditions such as high blood pressure, hypertension, joint and back pain, and even diabetes. We never realized we would start seeing benefits so quickly.

If you are reading this book, you or someone you know is considering weight-loss surgery. It's always scary when you start the contemplation and research. There are so many questions to answer and so many questions you don't even know you have yet. I want you to be comfortable and confident in your search. I want you to be armed with information and knowledge and set yourself up to be the best patient you can be. It's a scary step to take, but the more you know and understand, the more comfortable and reassuring it will be when you do make a choice.

As you contemplate having weight-loss surgery, do you think about it bringing happiness into your life? Do you have a wish list for your postoperative life? Have you longed for a particular lifestyle, but your weight has held you back?

When my husband and I started our journaling (see Chapter 5), we had our own wish list—I'm talking our basic wants. Individuals who have never been morbidly obese probably wouldn't find these to be things they would put on a wish list, but they were important to each of us. Things like:

- Walking without getting out of breath
- Getting in a car and being able to sit upright, without reclining the seat so far we felt we were driving from the backseat
- Wearing a seat belt without an extender
- Fitting into armchairs
- Riding in a plane or on an amusement park ride without worrying about not fitting
- Sitting in a restaurant booth and knowing there would be enough room
- Going to the movies and being able to sit comfortably in the seats
- Going into a bathroom and not having to use the handicap stall because it was larger
- Taking a nice hot bath and not having to get on my knees to get out
- Sitting on the floor and being able to get up without rolling over
- Crossing my legs
- Having a lap for my grandkids to sit on

- Grocery shopping without people checking out what's in our shopping cart
- Pushing a shopping cart and not having to lean on it for support
- Tying my shoes effortlessly
- Buying shoes in a normal width
- Wearing a shirt tucked in
- Wearing nonstretch pants
- Wearing shorts
- Buying clothes in sizes that don't have a letter attached (W, XXL)
- Hugging each other and being able to reach all the way around
- Having someone say "you're pretty" or "you're handsome" instead of saying "you sure would be pretty/handsome if you lost weight"

This list could go on and on, and I'm certain you have your own wants and wishes you could add. In fact, here are a few more from our chat boards:

- Walking anywhere no matter how long it takes
- Sitting in a lawn chair without being afraid to break it
- Sweating less
- Buying beautiful clothes
- Being smaller than my partner
- Wearing my partner's T-shirts to bed or to lounge in
- Wearing the robe at the spa or salon
- Being able to weigh on a regular household scale
- Sitting on the floor cross-legged
- Having energy to play with my kids and/or grandkids

Do you have your own wish list? Think about the things you miss, even if they would be insignificant to someone else. If it's important enough for you to be thinking about or wishing for, then it's an important part of your desire to succeed. You can write in your own top 10 list in the journal in Appendix B.

One way we build confidence and good momentum with people considering surgery is to help them imagine the ways their lives can improve. Think back to a time when you were smaller and healthier. Close your eyes, if you like, and return to that place. Can you remember what it was like? Or, if you were never in that place, can you imagine what it would be like?

Consider what it would mean to you to get out of the "high-risk" category and return to good health. What would change? Would you be able to cut back on medications or doctor visits? Is there someone whose mind you would put at ease about your health?

Also think about the ways you enjoyed and treasured life when you were healthier. Sometimes we all don't appreciate things until we lose them, and this could be looked at the same way. This is a second chance for life. What would you like to do with it?

Finally, make a wish list of whatever is important to you, small changes or big, past activities you have missed or new ones you want to try. Make it as long as you want. You can use the journal pages in Appendix B or your own journal.

After going through weight-loss surgery, you're going to find that new doors and new opportunities open up for you. Little did we know, for example, that doing something for our own health would turn into such a passion. Our own journey evolved from a small local support group into a message board, and that became a network of worldwide members who feel like family. Then the message board spawned a website. Then we began helping people start support groups. And then came speaking engagements.

This book isn't about us. It's about you. It's about you having the surgery. It's about you on maintenance. It's about your friends and family members who want to be part of the process and the success. It's about answering your questions or bringing up new questions for you to consider. This is a journey that is all about you and your understanding of this procedure. I firmly believe that you'll learn not only about this procedure but about yourself along the way as well. It's a new chapter in your life that comes with a whole new way of looking at and dealing with things you thought you knew instinctively, such as eating. I want to arm you with the right tools to make your story a success.

Dan and I talk with thousands upon thousands of people each month. Whether it's individuals in a local group or in a grocery line or at a speaking engagement, our support family grows exponentially. Our website continues to grow, and we want to continue to keep it fresh and informative as well. The message boards and outpouring of support from around the world is the most phenomenal thing. The success stories we hear every single day are encouraging and heartwarming, and it's a privilege to be a part of such a monumental time in so many people's lives. It's like sharing in the ultimate joys in your life over and over again, with thousands of your best friends.

In the following chapters, you're going to discover how you, too, can make a change for the better. You'll learn how to tell if the surgery is right for you, how to make the most out of the surgery, how to track your progress, and how to enjoy every weight-loss milestone of your exciting journey. I'll share what I've learned from working with thousands of weight-loss surgery patients and give you the information you need to reclaim your life. And you won't just hear from me, you'll hear from other patients as well—people just like you, who love their new life after weight-loss surgery.

I never thought we would equate weight loss to happiness or to smiling more, but I do. Dan and I both have always been positive, upbeat, fun-loving individuals, but we didn't realize how much we were missing out on until the weight started coming off. Today, we're blessed in more ways than just health. Our surgeries and our commitment to losing weight have been good for our hearts and souls, too. They have brought about so many changes in our lives. Happiness doesn't even begin to describe what we have experienced or continue to experience through each person we talk with. We share in their joy and happiness—it's contagious! We hope you catch what we have, and we hope you'll love being a big loser as much as we do, turning a negative into a positive and enjoying life again!

1

A New Life Is Waiting for You!

The day of our surgery was so exciting for my husband, Dan, and me. We do almost everything together, and this was no different: we chose to have weight-loss surgery at the same hospital with the same surgeon on the same morning. When we drove to the hospital, we didn't feel one shred of nervousness or fear, just plain excitement. I mean down-to-your-toes, spine-tingling, take-your-breath-away excitement. We had given up so much on account of our morbid obesity, but now we had the chance to start over. A whole new life was waiting just ahead of us. It was almost too much to believe that this was finally going to be the tool that would allow us to lose weight and to regain our health and our lives. After so many failed attempts, after letting ourselves down time and time again, we were confident this time was the right time. This time was the final time. This time was our time.

Our Story: Why We Chose Weight-Loss Surgery

Never in our wildest dreams had Dan and I thought we'd become "morbidly obese." We never imagined it could happen to us, but all of a sudden we realized we were struggling with even the simplest of tasks. Bending over and tying our shoes, for example, would leave us red-faced and out of breath. (If you are morbidly obese, you quickly learn to tie your shoes with one hand, on the side of your shoe, or you buy slip-on shoes or tennis shoes with Velcro.) I love relaxing in a nice hot bath, but that would mean rolling around in a slippery tub, trying to get onto my knees just to get out—another humiliation that deprived me of some of the small joys in everyday life.

And have you looked at clothing available for the obese and morbidly obese lately? Although a few designers actually provide decent-looking clothing in larger sizes, what are most designers thinking? "Let's make it in the shape of a tent and add BIG flowers or designs to it. That'll sure slim you down." Buying clothes in "normal" sizes became a thing of the past, and stretch pants became our clothing of choice, topped with big, baggy shirts. As my sister-in-law always says, "normal" is only a setting on the clothes dryer, and yet I missed the days when I could shop the ordinary aisles.

In addition to clothes, there were our closets, which were filled with such an array of sizes that we could have opened our own clothing store. What felt really bad was squeezing ourselves into too-tight clothes just to keep from facing the humiliation of going up in size, one more time.

The Restrictions on Our Lifestyle

If the clothing options weren't enough to scare us into losing weight, the personal restrictions set off all the alarms. We had brand-new bikes and beautiful places to ride, but our weight made riding for any length of time feel like torture. Besides, our own "seats" were now much wider than the actual bike seats—how could something as wide as that seat disappear so quickly when my rear end got on it?

Then there was the diminished lung capacity. Huffing and puffing and peddling weren't exactly our idea of a fun time. I can't even begin to imagine how comical we looked when trying to ride those poor, straining bicycles. We finally gave up because it was just too difficult—and even more embarrassing. There was no such thing as aerobic exercise any longer in our household. No longer did we go for long walks, or even short walks, for that matter. I felt out of breath after a slow walk to my car and got winded just crossing a room. I couldn't climb stairs without extreme joint pain, and I needed repeated stops to rest and catch my breath.

Dan and I loved swimming at the beach, but the thought of putting on a bathing suit was so repulsive that I hid my swimsuits. All I could imagine was the pointing, the stares, and the comments about a "beached whale sighting" if I appeared on the sand or coming out of the water. Any type of physical exertion became less and less of a priority, so we settled even deeper into our sedentary lifestyle and the habits of morbid obesity.

Meanwhile, the pounds kept piling up on us. Dan laughingly calls weight gain the furniture disease: where your chest finally drops into your drawers. We couldn't be getting bigger again, could we? Must be that our arms were getting shorter, because it was sure getting harder and harder to reach around each other.

We both woke up one day and realized we were in our forties and far from the fulfilling lives we should have been leading. Our kids were grown, and we were grandparents who were so out of shape we couldn't even play with our beautiful granddaughters.

We were letting this monster control us. How did two such strong, independent, intelligent individuals let this happen to themselves? That's what so many feel. How did they "let" this happen?

The Discrimination We Experienced

It wasn't just what we couldn't do anymore that made life so discouraging. It was also how people treated us, lumping us into a category of undesirables due to our size. We didn't have the flat abs or the toned arms and back. And so we were discriminated against, belittled, teased, chided, and tormented over our size.

One day, for example, I decided to stop in Victoria's Secret and do a little browsing. I typically stayed away from this type of store because the people who worked there tended to automatically turn up their noses, as if they would get fat just by touching me. But that day, no one else was in the store, so I went in. Shortly after I walked in, four or five other customers wandered in as well. All of them were waited on, but not once was I asked if I needed help. Finally, I became so aggravated that I went to the counter to seek assistance.

The clerks ignored me. Then they began to talk among themselves, three feet in front of me, as if I couldn't hear them. (Did they think that obesity affects the hearing?) One clerk commented to the other, "That one needs to go across the way to Lane Bryant. We don't have anything for someone like her." The other customers in the store heard this, and two actually began to laugh. It was worse than a slap in the face. This girl was standing there telling everyone within earshot that I wasn't worthy of basic human politeness just due to my size! Didn't she realize that I could have been shopping for someone else? Better yet, that it wasn't her place to make such terrible and hurtful judgments? I'd like to say this was a rare occurrence, but it was more the norm for someone living the morbidly obese life.

As if other people's insults weren't bad enough, we learned to heap this same abuse on ourselves. We spent countless hours scrutinizing every flaw we had—every roll or ripple, every wrinkle, sag, or bag. We could spot any and all imperfections without even looking closely.

The morbidly obese even learn to discriminate against themselves. Sometimes, this self-discrimination was due to very real concerns about not fitting into small areas. At restaurants or movie theaters, for example, seats might be too small. A friend of ours, Jamie, loved going out with friends for coffee or to restaurants. But as soon as someone invited her to such an outing, she'd drive over to the place to scope it out, to see if she'd be all right there. Were the chairs big enough? Was there enough space for her to move between the tables? Could she get in and out of the establishment without climbing stairs? If she had any doubt, she'd cancel the date. She didn't say why, she'd just cancel and live without.

Airplane trips offered other difficulties. Even with an extender, the seat belt could be too short or too tight. Some airlines have added more shame and humiliation by pulling us out of line to weigh us in front of everyone and declare us too heavy. Adding insult to injury, we have been charged for two seats each due to our size. Then there were the looks from strangers who were just hoping and praying they didn't have to sit next to us.

For some people, the situation gets desperate. The hostility and insults and their own hopelessness about their lives can even drive some morbidly obese people to suicide. That's not the norm, but it's certainly an indicator of how words can deeply affect people. Those same words, however, can also be the catalyst that helps people decide it's finally time to put a stop to all of this. Of course, it's just weight, which doesn't make you a bad or less-than-desirable person—you're just a larger person! There's nothing offensive about being larger. But we all know it is unhealthy, which makes finding a solution all the more important.

—————————— MAKING THE CONNECTION ——————————

Rachel's Story: I had two memorable plane rides. The first one was taken 30 days pre-op, when I couldn't fit into the seat. As if that weren't bad enough, I had to be embarrassed three times while asking for seat belt extenders. On top of that, I couldn't even put the tray table down, and I actually had to listen to two women argue loudly about who was going to have to get the "bad seat" next to me. The bad seat? I was relegated to being an undesirable?

Fast-forward to just one year later, and I was flying again. This time, the tray table went down, there was plenty of room left on the seat belt, and I could actually cross my legs. My husband even put me in the middle seat because I was now the "tiny one" and had plenty of room sitting between two people. As you can imagine, I cried on both trips: the first time out of anguish and the second out of joy!

Our Comorbidities

Although obesity stole so much that Dan and I enjoyed in life, we still weren't ready to try surgery. It just seemed so unknown, so extreme. Then one day, I realized I might lose Dan to obesity, too. We were seeing our primary care physician, and he said Dan had "comorbidities." Sounds deadly, doesn't it? (It is!) I went into panic mode. Was that the name of a disease? Is there a cure for it? How did we catch it? Is there a pill you can take?

Comorbidities are life-threatening, serious health issues and/or diseases that stem from carrying too much weight. We asked our doctor to explain some of the comorbidities. The first was sleep apnea, where you stop breathing hundreds of times in your sleep. Dan's snoring from sleep apnea was enough to scare anyone half to death. All I could do was pray for a few minutes

of quiet each night, although I certainly wasn't going to sleep
in another room. But as loud as his snoring was, it would scare
me when he wasn't snoring, because it meant he wasn't breathing. To keep Dan breathing, the doctor sent him home with a
BiPAP machine. I'm not sure which was worse, the sound of that
machine (kind of a Darth Vader effect) or the mask with the
long hose attached. Sometimes I didn't know if the machine was
helping Dan breathe or sucking the life right out of him.

Another comorbidity was GERD (gastroesophageal reflux
disease). We had thought that was just a little acid indigestion
that Dan had. All day. Every day. A third comorbidity was back,
hip, knee, ankle, and joint pain and swelling. This isn't sounding
good at all, is it? These are all comorbidities, aggravated by obesity, and there are a whole lot more, including the following.

Comorbidities Associated with Obesity

- High blood pressure
- Hypertension
- Gall bladder disease
- Shortness of breath
- Heart disease
- Diabetes
- High cholesterol
- Joint pain and swelling
- Sleep apnea
- GERD (reflux disease)

With so many comorbidities, and many of them aggravating
the others, our doctor was giving Dan a death sentence. As it
turns out, once a single comorbidity pops up, more may appear
in rapid succession.

Our biggest scare came with a trip to the orthopedic surgeon,
of all places. Unrelated to his comorbidities, Dan had hurt his

shoulder. When the surgeon began doing his exam, he pushed in on Dan's shins and his skin stayed indented almost two inches deep. Between that and some other signs, the doctor stopped the exam and insisted we go to a cardiologist. I don't mean that he asked us to schedule an appointment; I mean he made us leave his office and go straight to the heart doctor because Dan had the symptoms of congestive heart failure. The scariest part was that Dan's mother had died of congestive heart failure at the age of 53. Dan was about to turn 50. All I could think of was my precious husband dying—and all due to weight. A slow, painful progression of illnesses would lead to a senseless death sentence.

I was lucky enough not to suffer from comorbidities myself. My doctor liked to tell me I was "a healthy fat chick." But I knew that it was a matter of when—and not if—they would catch up to me.

The Surgery Has Worked for Us— and for Millions of Others, Too

Dan and I are exactly like the friends we've met through our website and at speaking engagements. Perhaps you see a bit of yourself in our story, too.

One of my favorite success stories is that of Stacey and Nick. Stacey and Nick share everything. They both even come from families where "big" is the norm and where family events are celebrated with tables groaning with food—and admonishments to clean their plates. They both developed tough outer skins to deflect the comments of total strangers and wicked senses of humor that helped them poke fun at themselves and beat others to the punch.

When Nick and Stacey met, they made a deal to try to be healthier. They tried various diets together, with no lasting suc-

HEALTH RISKS ASSOCIATED WITH OBESITY

If you are morbidly obese, here are some of the other health risks you may face:

- Angina, hypertension, and heart disease
- Asthma and other breathing/respiratory disorders
- Back pain
- Cancer
- Carpal tunnel syndrome
- Deep vein thrombosis
- Degenerative arthritis and osteoarthritis
- Depression and other psychosocial disorders
- Digestive and renal diseases
- Immobility
- Infertility and other reproductive/gynecological disorders
- Insulin resistance and diabetes
- Joint pain and other musculoskeletal disorders
- Leg swelling and varicose veins
- Liver disease
- Pancreatitis
- Skin infections
- Sleep apnea
- Stroke and other blood clots
- Ulcers
- Urinary stress incontinence

cess. Finally, they just gave up and decided to accept themselves and love their bodies. But there was always a question in Nick's mind about a procedure he'd heard of called gastric bypass surgery.

When Nick met Stacey, her older sister was in the process of obtaining insurance approval for the procedure. It sounded like a really good idea to Nick, but he kept his thoughts to himself. Stacey was adamant that it would not be an avenue she would ever consider, telling Nick the horror story of her mother.

In 1978, Stacey's mom underwent intestinal bypass surgery. Back then, doctors simply removed most of the small bowel and then sent the patient home with little or no instruction about living with this radically new digestive tract. Stacey's mom received no nutritional or psychological counseling to help her in her healing process. She walked out of the hospital hearing the words most fat people dream of hearing: "Go ahead, eat whatever you want, and you'll never gain a pound."

Eleven years later, she went to the doctor for mysterious abdominal bloating. Subsequent tests showed massive liver failure and critical vitamin deficiencies. Stacey's mother passed away shortly thereafter, ironically enough from malnutrition. On her deathbed, she made all her daughters promise to never undergo any sort of surgery for weight loss, no matter the advances in medicine. For Stacey, the issue of gastric bypass was closed.

At night, though, Nick began surfing the Internet and reading more and more about gastric bypass. He learned that many patients are cured of acid reflux disease, high blood pressure, and diabetes, all of which he had, and that the procedure was radically different from the operation that Stacey's mom had undergone. Nick joined a bunch of online groups for bypass patients and listened to many success stories. He finally confessed to Stacey that he was considering it, but the look of fear and horror on her face was enough to make him drop the subject.

Weeks later, Nick brought up the subject again. Stacey confessed that she had been doing research to dissuade Nick, but she realized that it might be a good thing for both of them. After a few false starts, they attended an informational seminar led by a gastric bypass surgeon, who took the time to explain the procedure in great detail. The doctor even sat with Stacey, hugging her when she related the story of her mother. His humanity and his success rate sealed the deal for both Nick and Stacey. They were going to have surgery.

Many medical tests, consults, and support group meetings later, the nurses wheeled Stacey away for her surgery. An hour later, she was done and recovering nicely. Two weeks later, she sat in the same waiting room while Nick had his surgery. One week later, they were walking around downtown Disney, sipping protein shakes and feeling like the luckiest people in the world.

Being able to whip out their "before" pictures is such a blast for them. The procedure has boosted their self-esteem and confidence. Nick feels better than he has felt in his entire adult life—his blood pressure is good, diabetes is a thing of the past, and acid reflux is a distant memory. Nick and Stacey both enjoy life now, instead of hiding from it.

One of the best things to come out of the surgery is the people they have met through their support group. Being able to keep each other motivated and abreast of the latest news in nutrition and health has been pivotal in their success as weight-loss surgery patients. Surgeons can perform the surgery on almost anyone, but the real success is keeping the weight off and remaining motivated. Surgery is only one part of the equation—motivation and careful attention to food and diet is another. Nick and Stacey work hard to get in enough protein and water each day, and they feel like a million bucks because of it.

The only negative thing is the impact all the new clothing has had on their checkbook. They have lost 287 pounds between the two of them and are not shy about clothes shopping. With both of them having the surgery, buying two complete new wardrobes

─────────── MAKING THE CONNECTION ───────────

Betsy's Story: I was 57 years old when I had my surgery. Before that time, I was out of breath all the time, and my physician was concerned I was a candidate for heart attack or stroke due to hypertension, high cholesterol, and asthma that was out of control. I could walk only when aided by a rolling walker.

I had so many worries and concerns about the surgery. Would my age inhibit my recovery? Would I have a safe and uneventful procedure? My worries were for naught, and all my prayers were answered. Not only did I lose 157 pounds (from a starting weight of 311 pounds) but my blood pressure, asthma, and cholesterol are now under control. Best yet, my mobility has returned, and I now walk, unaided, anywhere I desire. No more walker and no more shortness of breath—or any other medical problems, for that matter. I'm healthier than I've ever been as an adult. Not only was this the best decision I ever made, but I'm now also enjoying a healthy, active, unencumbered life filled with great days that possess unending possibilities.

---

has been pricey—but having to do it a couple of times before the weight loss settled in was a happy dilemma.

Their new goal is to complete their long-forgotten college degrees. Nick credits their newly positive self-image with giving them the confidence to try. Gastric bypass surgery saved their lives, and now they're finally living.

The Little Things That Make Life More Enjoyable

Before our surgeries, Dan and I were such big people that we could drive only big vehicles, large SUVs. When it was time to replace my vehicle after the surgery, I called the dealer as I had always done, and he sent me pictures of the different colors from which I could choose an equally large car. When I got to the dealership, though, I stopped to look at a Mustang on the showroom floor, shiny and brand new, the 1960s version. I'd always loved a Mustang. My heart just melted as I walked around and around it, petting it like it might follow me home. I dared to open the driver's-side door, and then it happened: I slid into the driver's seat. I mean I really slid in! I didn't have to be wedged in or pulled out. I could get in, get out, get in, get out without the least bit of trouble. Once I was in that car, however, I *didn't* get out until I'd driven it home!

Buying that car was fun, but it was *more* than fun. That day, I realized how my life was radically changing, how my efforts were worthwhile. That realization renewed my enthusiasm to stick with my new approach to food and health.

There were other successes. Our very first came before we even left the hospital. Our surgeon expected us to be up and walking the halls as part of our recovery, so we walked together. On those walks, we would pass a scale by the nurse's station. On the second day after surgery, I couldn't stand the suspense any longer and had to see what I weighed. I remember thinking, "I bet I've lost at least a couple of pounds." I eased myself on the scale. Most of the time, a step on the scale was not something worth sharing with Dan or anyone else. This time, though, a squeal slipped out, loud and clear. It was evidently louder than I realized because two nurses came running around the corner to see whether I had hurt myself. There I stood, beaming, and getting on and off that scale. I was thinking it *must* be broken because it said I'd lost 14 pounds! Granted, I know it was mostly fluid, but it was 14 pounds! The nurses began to laugh, and Dan just hugged me tight, with the IV pole in tow. I could tell already that the scale was going to become my new best friend during the weight-loss process.

One of my favorite stories is a tearjerker. It had been a couple of years since Dan and his brother, JT, had seen each other. We were just shy of the one-year anniversary of our surgeries, and we flew to Austin to visit Dan's family. JT agreed to pick us up at the airport, meeting us at the baggage carousel. Dan was leaning up against a column, and when he spotted his brother, he stood up straight and looked directly at him. All JT saw was some stranger staring him down, and it made him quite uncomfortable. About 10 feet in front of Dan, JT stopped in his tracks. His eyes filled with tears and he lunged at his brother for the biggest, longest hug. He grabbed him, hugged him, and held Dan out to look at him. He was shocked at how wonderful his brother looked. That moment of recognition and realization was such a beautiful and heartwarming sight.

One day, Dan and I were walking through a hardware store, and he picked up four 40-pound bags of salt for our water softener. With two bags in each hand, 80 pounds on each side, Dan struggled to walk. Suddenly he stopped, realizing that those heavy bags totaled 160 pounds, which was exactly the amount he had lost at that point. How could he have carried so much weight on his body all of those years? Dan said that moment made it even clearer for him that the decision to have gastric bypass had been the right choice for him. To this day, he will still stop and pick up similar bags, to remind himself of what 160 extra pounds felt like on his body.

As your weight comes off after the surgery, I encourage you, too, to seek out and enjoy all sorts of things that weren't possible for you before. It doesn't have to be something expensive, like a car. You might simply pass up the handicapped stall in the bathroom, choosing to use the regular one instead. Or maybe you'll wrap a regular towel around you—and it stays up! Perhaps it'll be wearing clothes that don't have a W or an XXXL on the tag. Or your child lays her head in your lap and you think, "I have a lap! Where did *that* come from?"

Start Your New Life Now

There's no price you can put on your health or your happiness. If you are like many, the weight comes on gradually. And you may not realize that as the weight piles on, you begin to close off more and more. You may stop doing things you loved or stop seeing people you loved because you don't feel good about yourself.

Fortunately, you can reclaim that lost feeling of happiness. Actually, you can replace it with an entirely new feeling of elation. It's almost like discovering life all over again. Everything is new and fresh and is just sitting there waiting for you to tackle it. Even years after surgery, you'll still find activities you can do that you used to keep in the "can't do" part of your brain. With being happier and having more fun comes a more active lifestyle.

Dan and I know. After feeling like we were chained down for so many years, now we could get out and do things without feeling self-conscious or getting winded or worrying we wouldn't fit. This change seemed like it started almost overnight, even more emotionally than physically from that first day. We were both filled with so much excitement and enthusiasm for what was ahead. After all the years of yo-yo dieting, we both knew this was finally the answer for us.

Happy stories and life changes like this occur almost daily. This surgery, this incredible tool, was the key to unlocking our prison that we called obesity, and it has been the key for millions of others as well. In Chapter 2, you'll discover the facts about weight-loss surgery—especially whether your current situation makes you a good candidate for the procedure—as well as address any fears you (or your family) might have about it. That information will help you decide whether weight-loss surgery might be the key to your new life, too!

2

Researching Weight-Loss Surgery—and Making Your Decision

Have any of these thoughts crossed your mind?

- Am I crazy (or am I giving up) by considering surgery to lose weight?
- How do I know if this surgery is right for me?
- How will my life change after weight-loss surgery?

- Will I miss my old way of life after the surgery?
- Will I ever eat again?

Questions race around your mind as you start thinking about the procedure. Your emotions become akin to a roller-coaster ride with ups, downs, twists, and turns at high speeds. One minute you are at the apex and surveying the path ahead, filled with excitement and anticipation. The next thing you know, you're flying so fast on the track that your stomach is jumping into your throat and your heart is racing 90 miles per hour. You have many questions and concerns about such a drastic decision. Where do you start? What do you do? What do you ask? Whom do you ask? Where do you look? Like most prospects, weight-loss surgery is scariest when you don't understand it or know what to expect.

You will likely have a million questions and concerns running through your mind, and they'll start coming at you even faster after you begin researching. These questions and concerns are understandable and perfectly normal. If you weren't apprehensive about such a big decision, then *that* would be something to be concerned about.

This chapter starts you on the path to making a decision. Here, you will learn the facts, get answers to the most frequently asked questions, brush your fears aside, and feel confident in your decision, whatever that decision is.

Are You a Candidate for Weight-Loss Surgery?

Whether you're a candidate for weight-loss surgery is something for you and your doctor to determine, but there are some basic questions that can guide you. If you answer yes to any of the following, you could be a candidate for weight-loss surgery:

- Are you at least 90 to 100 pounds over your ideal body weight?
- Do you have a body mass index (BMI) of 40 or more?
- Do you have a BMI of 35 or more and experience any combination of at least two of the following: high blood pressure or hypertension, diabetes, GERD or acid reflux, joint paint due to excessive weight, or fatty liver (nonalcoholic)?

If so, read on.

Checking Your BMI

Calculating BMI is one of the first things you do to determine if weight-loss surgery is right for you. Some think of BMI as the same as body fat, but they are not the same. Body mass index is a correlation between your height and weight that is associated with your body fat and health risk. A BMI of 25 is considered obese. If your BMI is over 40 or have a BMI of 35 along with at least two comorbidities, you're a candidate for weight-loss surgery. If your BMI is 30 and you have serious comorbidities (see Chapter 1), you may also qualify under some extreme guidelines. Under these guidelines, at least 15 million people in the United States now qualify, and the true number may be 20 million or higher.

To manually calculate your BMI, you're going to need a scale, a measuring tape or other means of measuring your height, a notepad, a pen, and a calculator.

How to Calculate Your BMI

1. Begin with your weight and write it down.
2. Measure your height in inches and write it down.
3. In your notepad and using your calculator, square your height by multiplying your height in inches by your height in inches. For example, someone 6 feet tall would be 72 inches, so multiply: $72 \times 72 = 5,184$.

Table 2.1 Body Mass Index

Height (inches)	Normal						Overweight					Obese										Extreme Obesity														
BMI	19	20	21	22	23	24	25	26	27	28	29	30	31	32	33	34	35	36	37	38	39	40	41	42	43	44	45	46	47	48	49	50	51	52	53	54
												Body Weight (pounds)																								
58	91	96	100	105	110	115	119	124	129	134	138	143	148	153	158	162	167	172	177	181	186	191	196	201	205	210	215	220	224	229	234	239	244	248	253	258
59	94	99	104	109	114	119	124	128	133	138	143	148	153	158	163	168	173	178	183	188	193	198	203	208	212	217	222	227	232	237	242	247	252	257	262	267
60	97	102	107	112	118	123	128	133	138	143	148	153	158	163	168	174	179	184	189	194	199	204	209	215	220	225	230	235	240	245	250	255	261	266	271	276
61	100	106	111	116	122	127	132	137	143	148	153	158	164	169	174	180	185	190	195	201	206	211	217	222	227	232	238	243	248	254	259	264	269	275	280	285
62	104	109	115	120	126	131	136	142	147	153	158	164	169	175	180	186	191	196	202	207	213	218	224	229	235	240	246	251	256	262	267	273	278	284	289	295
63	107	113	118	124	130	135	141	146	152	158	163	169	175	180	186	191	197	203	208	214	220	225	231	237	242	248	254	259	265	270	278	282	287	293	299	304
64	110	116	122	128	134	140	145	151	157	163	169	174	180	186	192	197	204	209	215	221	227	232	238	244	250	256	262	267	273	279	285	291	296	302	308	314
65	114	120	126	132	138	144	150	156	162	168	174	180	186	192	198	204	210	216	222	228	234	240	246	252	258	264	270	276	282	288	294	300	306	312	318	324
66	118	124	130	136	142	148	155	161	167	173	179	186	192	198	204	210	216	223	229	235	241	247	253	260	266	272	278	284	291	297	303	309	315	322	328	334
67	121	127	134	140	146	153	159	166	172	178	185	191	198	204	211	217	223	230	236	242	249	255	261	268	274	280	287	293	299	306	312	319	325	331	338	344
68	125	131	138	144	151	158	164	171	177	184	190	197	203	210	216	223	230	236	243	249	256	262	269	276	282	289	295	302	308	315	322	328	335	341	348	354
69	128	135	142	149	155	162	169	176	182	189	196	203	209	216	223	230	236	243	250	257	263	270	277	284	291	297	304	311	318	324	331	338	345	351	358	365
70	132	139	146	153	160	167	174	181	188	195	202	209	216	222	229	236	243	250	257	264	271	278	285	292	299	306	313	320	327	334	341	348	355	362	369	376
71	136	143	150	157	165	172	179	186	193	200	208	215	222	229	236	243	250	257	265	272	279	286	293	301	308	315	322	329	338	343	351	358	365	372	379	386
72	140	147	154	162	169	177	184	191	199	206	213	221	228	235	242	250	258	265	272	279	287	294	302	309	316	324	331	338	346	353	361	368	375	383	390	397
73	144	151	159	166	174	182	189	197	204	212	219	227	235	242	250	257	265	272	280	288	295	302	310	318	325	333	340	348	355	363	371	378	386	393	401	408
74	148	155	163	171	179	186	194	202	210	218	225	233	241	249	256	264	272	280	287	295	303	311	319	326	334	342	350	358	365	373	381	389	396	404	412	420
75	152	160	168	176	184	192	200	208	216	224	232	240	248	256	264	272	279	287	295	303	311	319	327	335	343	351	359	367	375	383	391	399	407	415	423	431
76	156	164	172	180	189	197	205	213	221	230	238	246	254	263	271	279	287	295	304	312	320	328	336	344	353	361	369	377	385	394	402	410	418	426	435	443

Source: Adapted from *Clinical Guidelines on the Identification, Evaluation, and Treatment of Overweight and Obesity in Adults: The Evidence Report.*

4. Divide your weight (in total pounds) by your height squared. For example, 400 lb ÷ 5,184 = .07716.
5. Multiply that answer by 703. For example, 77.16 × 703 = 54.24 BMI.

There's another way to calculate BMI, and either is correct. I'm listing the second way here, in case your physician does it this way:

1. Multiply your weight in pounds by 703. For example, 400 × 703 = 281,200.
2. Divide by your height in inches. For example, 281,200 ÷ 72 = 3905.56.
3. Divide by your height in inches again. For example, 3905.56 ÷ 72 = 54.24.

An even simpler method is to use a BMI chart, such as the one shown in Table 2.1. Find your height in inches down the left side and follow it across until you find your weight. Along the top of the chart, you'll find your BMI.

You can also find websites with free BMI calculators, where you just plug in your height and your weight and it instantly provides your BMI. Some sites are:

- bariatricedge.com
- nhlbisupport.com/bmi

Checking Your Willingness to Stop the Cycle of Overeating

What gets many of us in trouble is our emotional attachment to food. We eat not for our bodies but for our feelings. We all have to eat enough to fuel our bodies and minds. But many of us keep on eating when our body has what it needs, whether from

WEIGHT-LOSS SURGERY AND TYPE 2 DIABETES

In the future, weight-loss surgery may no longer be reserved for only the morbidly obese. A 2008 article in *The Journal of the American Medical Association* found that patients who had recently been diagnosed with type 2 diabetes and were obese—but who did not necessarily meet the BMI standards for morbid obesity currently required by insurance companies—saw marked improvements in their diabetes conditions compared to patients who were given only weight-loss counseling and diabetes medications.

Of the 60 patients studied, 73 percent of those who had weight-loss surgery no longer had any sign of type 2 diabetes, compared to 13 percent of those who did not undergo surgery. And this makes sense, given that type 2 diabetes is often triggered by obesity. The weight-loss surgery group, not surprisingly, also lost substantially more weight—nearly 21 percent of their body weight, versus less than 2 percent in the nonsurgery group.

This study—when supplemented by additional studies and if accepted by the medical insurance community—could lead to a relaxing of the BMI guidelines for weight-loss surgery. Currently, a BMI of 40 is the cutoff for surgery, unless comorbidities (including type 2 diabetes) exist, when the standard is relaxed to 35. But 22 percent of the diabetics in this study had BMIs under 35, currently making them ineligible for insurance coverage for the surgery, which can cost up to $25,000. If your BMI is less than 35 and you have type 2 diabetes, keep checking with your physician and insurance company to determine whether you become eligible in the future.

boredom, anxiety, or trying to make up for something missing in our lives.

Some people "graze" all day, while others clean their plate just because it's there. Some eat absentmindedly through movies or television, while others just keep eating dessert until there's nothing left. And how many times have you tried to smooth over your sorrows with a bowl of ice cream or a bag of chips or cookies? All of this is what's known as emotional eating, and the list of places and times for it is endless. It's eating for comfort, solace, pleasure, and company, to fill the isolation.

That kind of eating is the big risk to weight-loss success, even after surgery. It's true that surgery can take away the hunger, but it's no guarantee. Surgery can also make it very uncomfortable to overeat. Together, those two changes usually lead to dramatic results in the first months, and those dramatic results can renew your pride and confidence, giving you the encouragement you need to keep losing weight.

But even more important is a long-term emotional change from a life centered on food to a life centered on other things. I cannot stress enough the importance of getting your head to a new place. Weight-loss surgery is an amazing tool, but it's stomach surgery, not brain surgery. The stomach of an obese person is not diseased, and the surgery is not a cure. Rather, the surgery

---

MAKING THE CONNECTION

Dave Speaks About Emotional Eating: I am a big sweets eater, and my portions are way out of control. . . . I eat not because I am hungry but because I want or I need to pass time with food. I very rarely feel hunger; I just go from this to that, eating all day.

creates the opportunity to make the changes in your mind, your heart, and your habits that will lead to a new and healthier life. Unless you work with your brain and heart and soul as well, no stomach-changing tool can work in the long term.

This is so important it bears repeating: weight-loss surgery is a *tool* and it's all in how you use the tool that makes this procedure truly effective. If you had eating disorders before surgery, you're still going to have them after surgery. Are you an emotional eater? A stress eater? A compulsive overeater or a binge eater? Did you know that there's only a tiny difference between being a compulsive overeater and a binge eater? These issues won't go away simply by having surgery. If these issues sound like the ones you struggle with, get help from a counselor who specializes in eating disorders *before* undergoing surgery.

If you have a hammer, you can either build something big and wonderful with that hammer or you can tear something down and destroy it. It's the same concept with this great tool. You can maximize this tool and improve your habits and your lifestyle. But remember that this is a lifelong commitment, not a quick fix; it's definitely not the easy way out.

Family Issues

In your process of sorting through information and emotions, there may be people in your life who try to convince you to try dieting just one more time. Or you may try to convince yourself of this! We certainly went through these questions, but we ultimately realized that dieting hadn't worked for us those many times before, so why on earth, we thought, would it be any different this time? Losing the weight was never the real problem. Keeping it off and making it livable was.

But there are other concerns of family and friends that may be even more pressing. Is the procedure really safe? What if something goes wrong—what will happen to your children or other loved ones? Or maybe you have fears or concerns along the lines of what your friends or family will do without you. I don't mean as in losing you from gastric bypass surgery, but in terms of losing you to the issues connected with morbid obesity. Your parents, siblings, significant other, children, and friends may all be as connected to your obesity as you are. Some of them may challenge your decisions and doubt your choices. I address the issue of family and friends in more depth in Chapter 3.

Facing Fears: Our Story

When Dan and I were first contemplating weight-loss surgery, we set out to arm ourselves with as much information as possible, because that was going to be our only way of making an educated decision. Dan and I had had very different experiences when it came to surgery. I'd been under the knife a few times before, but this would be Dan's maiden surgery voyage. By the time we had ours scheduled, he was so well prepared and so excited that he wanted to be the one to go first. We were like two kids racing to get there first because we just couldn't wait to start this journey! But until that point, it took a lot of soul-searching plus research, research, and more research to weigh our options and decide whether surgery was the right answer for us.

Dan and I had seen bits and pieces of information on gastric bypass over the years. Every time we did, we would think about it and then file it in the backs of our minds. We would have conversations here and there, and then we would delve into more research. I'm relentless about due diligence, and we weren't going to take this lightly. After enough research, we started thinking about it seriously and talked with our primary care physician, but we were nervous.

Over the course of a couple of years, spending hours and hours on research, we kept coming up with horror stories and more reasons to worry. It was enough to scare anyone away from the surgery. But why was so much of the information so negative? And how had this surgical procedure managed to grow through the years if it was so bad and dangerous? Were we afraid of the surgery itself? Or of the horror stories that seemed to pop up from everyone? Didn't there have to be some good for this procedure to have been around for more than 50 years?

When we dug a little deeper, we saw a pattern. The majority of the negative stories about weight-loss surgery tended to come from people who were not or never had been obese, much less morbidly obese. Nor had the majority of reporters or writers, whose work we were reading, experienced weight-loss surgery themselves. As we slowly found the answers that put our fears to rest, we realized how important it would be to have good information for the people who really need it. Since then, we've talked to tens of thousands of people and heard from even more from around the world, and we've found that many of the questions and worries seem to be universal.

Answering Frequently Asked Questions

Before our surgery, Dan and I spent hours on end poring over websites and brochures and information from doctors, psychologists, nutritionists, message boards, and bariatric centers all around the world. We scoured bookstores, which turned up very little that we wanted to know. We found some technical-type books, but few, if any, dealt with life after surgery.

There are so many details to consider and so many pressing questions:

- How do I know which surgery is right?
- How much will insurance cover?

—————————— MAKING THE CONNECTION ——————————

Gilat Shares Her Emotions: In the past couple of days, I'm feeling more anxiety than ever. I'm scared to death. I'm scared of complications. I'm scared I will *not* lose the weight, and I'm starting to doubt my decision to have the surgery. As I read through my journal, I read my thoughts of and pains of being fat. I read it like it was someone else, another person who knew what she was getting herself into. I'm so anxious about what is going to happen.

I had another surgery some years earlier, and I don't think I was that scared then. After reading about another guy in the group, I decided to write down my fears, too. It felt better because my fears looked less serious and some even seemed silly to me when I read them again. I am *not* afraid of my surgeon or the facility. I am *definitely* ready to change my life and make an effort to succeed using this amazing tool. I also researched this so thoroughly that I feel I could be a consultant on the topic. I've been wasting my life, obese, for too many years. *I am ready.*

- Once I choose my surgery and surgeon, what can I expect?
- What should I ask the surgeon?
- Will I live through this? (And the corollary: Will I live if I don't have the surgery?)
- Will I miss my old foods?
- How do I wade through all the information and make a decision?

The following sections answer these main questions. Chapters 5 through 8 also deal with life after weight-loss surgery. In addition to the answers you'll find on the following pages, we encourage you to do your own research. An informed patient is a better patient, and the more you know before surgery, the better prepared you'll be to make the most of it! Be proactive about your decision and your care. It's your life, and no one cares about it the way you do.

There are many great sources for information. The American Society of Metabolic and Bariatric Surgery (asmbs.org) is the cornerstone for accurate information and answers regarding weight-loss surgery. Other sites, such as BariatricEdge (bariatricedge.com) and the Obesity Action Coalition (obesityaction.org), are a wealth of information, education, and answers. At these sites you'll find information from experts such as surgeons along with statistics, procedures, expectations, history, and additional research sources. You cannot be too educated or too prepared! Every bit of knowledge will aid you in making that right decision and feeling confident about your choice.

Which Surgery Is Right for Me?

You can only answer this question in consultation with a doctor. Despite the many surgeries with their different and often confusing names, however, there are only a few important differences to understand. Weight-loss surgery works by two methods, which are sometimes combined:

■ **Lap band surgery:** Laparoscopic adjustable gastric banding (better known as lap band) is a purely restrictive method in which the surgeon implants a ring or band to squeeze the stomach, so it holds less food and feels full faster.

■ **Gastric bypass surgery:** This is a procedure in which the surgeon removes part of the stomach, reattaching it further down the small intestine (thereby bypassing part of the small intestine). It is performed either laparoscopically or by way of open incision. The laparoscopic procedure typically involves six small incisions versus the open procedure, which requires one long, much more extensive incision. The medical name for this procedure is Roux-en-Y.

For many, lap band is a temporary solution to a permanent problem. While you now have a smaller pouch to replace that large stomach and have to eat smaller portions, those smaller portions could easily be milk shakes, ice cream, cookies, candy bars, and more. This means that not only would you *not* develop healthy eating habits but you would regain the weight you'd lost as a result of ingesting foods that are high in calories but of little or no nutritional value.

With gastric bypass, the typical patient can (and usually does) have an adverse effect known as dumping (see Chapter 4) to a variety of foods, ranging from sugary items to foods the system doesn't or won't tolerate. These foods, or the amount or the speed with which you eat them, can result in the pouch rejecting them and dumping into your small intestine. Tolerance levels vary by patient and by such issues as food type, doneness, density, moisture content, and a plethora of other variances. There's no one checklist of foods to stay away from. Sure there are better choices than others, but you can still have some issues when it comes to your body accepting even healthy foods.

Most people will attest that dumping is an unpleasant experience of varying degrees, but it is a valuable tool for the long term. After experiencing dumping a few times, you learn to make the necessary adjustments to avoid it. Dumping is a catalyst that aids you in learning to make different, healthier choices and develop better eating habits.

Gastric bypass is the procedure Dan and I chose and what we focus on in this book. However, the information we discuss is considered by many to be equally helpful to patients who are considering different versions of weight-loss surgery from ours.

Will Insurance Pay for the Procedure?

Many insurance companies pay for gastric bypass, but coverage varies greatly by company, inclusions in individual company policies, the state where the insurance is based, and more. Some of the standard items expected when qualifying through your insurance are as follows:

- Proof of a six-month supervised weight-loss attempt administered by a medical professional, such as your primary care physician
- Meeting the BMI guidelines of 40 (or 35 and at least two comorbidities); some insurance companies, on a case-by-case basis, will take a BMI as low as 30 with extensive comorbidities
- Referral by your primary care physician; some insurance companies require you to obtain a referral from your primary care physician prior to approval
- Psychological evaluation
- Nutrition counseling
- Preliminary lab work (a list provided by your surgeon)
- Preliminary screenings, such as sleep study, chest X-rays, gall bladder sonogram, stress tests, or whatever else is deemed necessary by your insurance company

While this list may look long, most of these tasks can be accomplished fairly quickly, other than the six-month supervised diet attempt, of course. The purpose of these tests is to ascertain that you are in the best physical and mental state, given your current weight, to withstand major surgery and the changes that will occur afterward.

I look at it this way: if they find anything wrong, it's far better to address it before surgery than when you're on an operating table. Give yourself the best possible head start and take these steps to heart. They're all in your best interest.

What Can I Expect from the Surgeon and the Surgery?

When you start investigating weight-loss surgery, one of the steps is to attend a surgery seminar. These seminars are typically free, and most bariatric centers provide them in a group setting. You will learn information on the procedure and what to expect from that center's particular program. Attending one or more of these sessions gives you an opportunity to hear and see what a particular surgeon does, as well as to discuss questions or concerns. This is an enlightening time and usually puts the process into fast-forward for you.

Most surgeons take you through a full description of the surgical procedure. Many potential patients don't realize that their new stomach pouch will be reduced from the size of a football to approximately the size of an egg. With diminished stomach capacity, you will learn to appreciate good-quality food choices so you get maximum benefits.

After surgery, your particular bariatric center will give you guidelines for an eating plan to carry you through the stages. Each center and surgeon is different—there is no single right program. There are better, more healthy choices, but there isn't one concrete "this is the only way" eating plan for post-op. You always, however, want to follow your surgeon's instructions.

We have found many commonalities in the early stages and weeks of eating plans. The first week is typically something along the lines of clear liquids, such as clear broth, 100 percent fruit juices, 100 percent fruit juice frozen bars (no sugar), noncarbonated water, no-sugar drinks, decaffeinated drinks, and protein drinks. When moving into the next stage, typically things like cream soups are added, even lobster bisque or pureed clam chowder. Finally, you'll be able to eat soft solid foods or pureed versions of solid foods.

Even in the first week, when you're on broth, go for flavor. At every stage of recovery and discovery, it's important to feed the senses and not just fill the void (that is, your new pouch). If you don't feed your head while you're refueling your body, you'll have a tendency to want to graze. Grazing usually occurs when you're looking for "something" to satisfy that missing taste. And that "something" is flavor. Be sure to give it to yourself. Before our surgeries, Dan and I planned ahead, cooked our own broths, and froze them (see Appendix A for recipes).

What Questions Should I Ask My Surgeon?

Most potential patients are surprised to find that the seminar is their first encounter with their surgeon; their second encounter is as they are finished with all the testing and ready for paperwork to be submitted to insurance. To maximize your surgeon's availability to you, you may want to start a list of questions. If you can't or don't get all your questions answered when you attend the seminar, start a new list for when you meet with your surgeon in his or her office for the final consultation. I've included a list of questions you might want to get answered during the seminar.

Seminar Questions

- Which procedure does the surgeon perform? For example, laparoscopic Roux-en-Y, open Roux-en-Y, lap band? We're constantly amazed by how many patients get all the way to having surgery and don't know what procedure they're having. Recovery times, risks for infection, and long-term success rates vary by which procedure you are having.
- How many procedures has the surgeon performed?

- How long has the surgeon been practicing?
- Is the bariatric program a Center of Excellence (COE)? Some insurance companies will pay for procedures only if they are performed through a Center of Excellence. Centers that have received this designation from the American Society of Metabolic and Bariatric Surgery (ASMBS) have exhibited high surgical skills, high quality of care, and low rates of complications. It's a stringent process to receive this designation, which is the ASMBS attempt to ensure the highest quality of surgical excellence.
- Has the surgeon him- or herself obtained the Center of Excellence standing? This is important because a surgeon can be part of a COE without personally having contributed to the rating.
- How long does the surgeon typically take to perform the procedure?
- What is the average hospital stay?
- How much time does the surgeon recommend that you take off work?
- Does the surgeon or center have any special eating plan that is required prior to surgery? For example, some require patients to be on an all-liquid diet for days or weeks before the surgery, while others may require a high-protein eating plan (to shrink the size of the liver).
- Is any weight loss required prior to surgery? Some programs require the patient to lose a minimal amount of weight to prove their seriousness and commitment. This is not a standard requirement, though.
- Is there a maximum weight cut-off the surgeon has where he or she will no longer do laparascopic Roux-en-Y and would switch to open Roux-en-Y? If you don't know the difference and need to know, ask that question, too.
- Does the surgeon hand stitch or staple the new smaller pouch? Or both? Each method has its advantages and disad-

vantages, and you'll want to speak to your surgeon about the different procedures and outcomes.

- Has the surgeon had problems with leaks in patients? A leak is a void in the pouch wall that allows fluid into the abdominal cavity. Most surgeons test for these while you're still in surgery, but it's important to know whether your surgeon has had cases of leaks discovered after surgery. Leaks require a return visit to surgery.

- How many leak tests does the surgeon do and when? Many surgeons do a test in the operating room and again the following day via a procedure known as a barium swallow.

- Has the surgeon had major complications? Were the complications directly related to the surgery itself or to the patient's health?

- Has the surgeon had any deaths specifically related to the procedure? If so, how many and what were the circumstances?

- If you're a smoker, does the surgeon require a specific time frame to quit? Does he or she do nicotine testing prior to surgery? (I cannot stress enough how critical it is you stop smoking as soon as you make the decision to have surgery!)

- How soon after surgery will you be up and walking?

- How soon after surgery before you're allowed to drive?

In addition to getting your questions answered, how do you get comfortable with a surgeon you have met only in a group setting and then once again just before surgery? Most people want to build a rapport with their surgeon before moving forward. For us, to be expected to be so trusting seemed like a lot to ask when we were first starting out. But we also now see the point. By having all your files, tests, and evaluations in front of him or her, your surgeon has the full picture of your health and any possible risks or obstacles that may need to be addressed.

If you've never had surgery, you might also want to ask other weight-loss surgery patients what their experiences were and for suggestions on what would have made them more comfortable. Your surgeon's support group, an online support group, or a message board are great sources for this info as well (see Chapter 4).

Is Weight-Loss Surgery Dangerous?

Surgery is surgery. Whether it's having your tonsils out or having a face-lift or removing an appendix, even the most routine surgeries carry some risk. These risks are greater for people who are overweight, because sleep apnea and other comorbidities (see Chapter 1) increase the risks from anesthesia. The published mortality figures range from 0.5 percent to 1 percent of weight-loss surgeries, but ask your surgeon about his or her specific mortality rate. You aren't as concerned with national averages as you are with those of the person who will actually be performing your procedure—this goes for mortality as well as for other risks.

The risk factors of weight-loss surgery vary from surgeon to surgeon, which means there are endless variables—surgeon experience, patient health, and patient age are just a few examples. On a national average, according to the ASMBS:

Assessing the risks of surgical treatment of obesity involves operative [during the surgery], perioperative [just after the surgery] and long term [long after the surgery] complications. Available published series report that the immediate operative mortality rate for both vertical banded gastroplasty and Roux-en-Y gastric bypass is relatively low. Morbidity [that is, the presence of illness] in the early postoperative period, i.e., wound infections, dehiscence [opening of a wound closed in surgery], leaks from staple breakdown, stomal stenosis [a narrowing of the opening or outlet of the stomach pouch], marginal ulcers, various pulmonary problems, and deep thrombophlebitis [inflammation and blood clot in a vein] may be as high as ten percent or more. Splenectomy [surgery on the spleen] is necessary in 0.3% of patients to control operative bleeding. However, the aggregate risk of the most serious complications of gastrointestinal leak and deep venous thrombosis is less than one percent.

As you'll see for yourself, when you review the risks, weight-loss surgery has a similar risk list to other elective surgeries—and those surgeries probably will *not* change your life!

Indeed, for most morbidly obese people it's dangerous *not* to have the surgery. Comorbidities (see Chapter 1) only worsen as you grow older and become less active, and the risks from those are serious. Not getting to a healthy weight is likely, over time, to leave you terribly sick or with serious health issues. That's why so many insurance plans (and now Medicare) cover the procedure. Obesity is a disease and has to be treated as such. This is one chronic disease that is preventable or curable when we find the right tools for us individually. Left unattended, it can lead to almost certain death.

Will I Be Able to Eat My Favorite Foods?

Maybe, maybe not. There are foods you will probably never eat again, but you will also quickly lose your taste for them. You will, however, be able to eat plenty of delicious foods again—have no fear! One of the most common myths is that once you have weight-loss surgery, you'll live a dull gastronomic life. Chapter 5 gives you all the specifics on how you'll eat, but the bottom line is this: you'll eat tiny meals (which, because of the size of your

SORTING THROUGH FRIGHTENING STORIES

For a while in the 1980s and 1990s, success almost spoiled weight-loss surgery. An influx of inexperienced surgeons started to do the procedure to "cash in" on the trend. The combination of inexperienced bariatric surgeons with obese patients who had special health needs added up to a dangerous situation. Unfortunately, in those early years, there were a few highly publicized deaths and malpractice cases. These few incidents tarnished the reputation of a procedure that is otherwise well established and safe. Horror stories began circulating and still do. There never fails to be the friend who knew someone, or heard of someone, yet specific names and dates tend to fail those recalling these stories. For some reason, it's human nature to remember the bad. But the truth is that the success stories far, far, far exceed any negatives that may have occurred.

pouch, will fill you up) that are high in protein, and you'll sip lots and lots of fluids throughout each day.

Your tastes will change from the very first day, and you'll be surprised at how extreme some of these changes may be. Things you loved before may become completely disgusting to you. For example, Dan and I were major soda drinkers before surgery. We each drank a case or more of carbonated drinks every single day. It's a wonder we had stomachs left from all the acid! Before the surgery, one of our biggest fears was missing those colas. But not only did we *not* miss them, it didn't take long for us to become hooked on water. Who would have believed we could make that change, that quickly? But we came to know that our soda drinking was an addiction we had, and we were glad to kick the habit.

Not only did I love my colas, but at a restaurant, I would look at the dessert menu before I even chose my entree. I would make room for whatever luscious, delectable, ooey, gooey confection I selected. From the very first day of surgery, though, I lost that taste for sweets. I don't mean just a little, either. On a scale of 1 to 100, if something was a 1 on the sweetness scale before, it was 100 on the post-op scale. The flavors were so heightened it was almost inconceivable that I was ever able to eat such things before. Based on the feedback I've gotten in support groups and on the Web, this experience is quite common after weight-loss surgery. After surgery, my old favorite foods just didn't hold that same place in my heart (or should I say, my blocked arteries!) that they did before. Now, the desire for dessert has been replaced by a genuine taste for fruit or other healthy choices.

Do we miss particular foods? No way! We still eat out, and no matter where we travel, we find healthy, delicious things to eat. Do we feel deprived? No. Because of the surgery, we don't have enough room to digest presurgery portions. We feel full more quickly, but we also appreciate and enjoy our food more.

Although I lost my taste for my favorite colas and desserts, Dan and I still make a point of steering clear of trigger foods— those foods that we always overindulge in, even when we don't mean to. If you know a particular food is a trigger for you, walk away from it. Don't bring it in the house. Don't test the waters. Assume it's going to make you dump (see Chapter 4), and just hold onto that thought.

As you contemplate weight-loss surgery, I cannot stress enough how important it is to work on your eating habits, both physical and emotional. Make sure you develop new healthy habits that will carry you through for a lifetime. (See Chapter 5 for more information on how to develop healthier eating habits after surgery.)

How Can I Decide What to Do?

To help you make a decision, you need to get your fears out in the open, while also reviewing your research. To start, make a three-column list and follow the instructions in the next four sections. You can write your answers in the journal pages in the back of the book or in your own journal.

This is a great tool for controlling your fears—or at least keeping them in check! Keep in mind, however, that this list is yours and applies only to you. It needs to reflect your thoughts, not anyone else's.

Column 1: List Your Fears About Obesity. One column is your being-fat fears. List your aches and pains and how they keep changing. List how they limit your life. List how you think they'll continue to increasingly limit you or even end your life early. Do you see the road ahead filled with fatigue, poor health, high blood pressure, heart issues, possible stroke, and more due to morbid obesity? (You may want to flip to Chapter 1 for a list of comorbidities and other health problems.) Does obesity limit your everyday activities and your interaction with friends and family? Does it keep you from performing to your fullest potential on your job? Choose whatever factors matter to you. It can be any and all details or issues, large and small, that matter to you. Consider this list a release of all those things you wouldn't share with someone else, but you need to be brutally honest with the person who matters most: you. Remember, it's about you and the questions or concerns you have. There are no right or wrong answers. Once complete, you'll see it as a road map guiding you where you need to go.

Column 2: List Your Fears About Having the Surgery. The next column on your list is your having-surgery fears. This one can be tricky because you may not even realize what it is you are afraid of. Is it that a virtual stranger will have you on an operating table and change your life forever? While you've researched the doctor to the best of your ability, it's not like you've been in the operating room watching him or her doing these procedures over and over.

You may also fear what the surgery is going to feel like. Most people find that they barely remember getting into the operating room, and they sure aren't aware of anything else going on, but if this is one of your fears or questions, write it down. You may also wonder what happens when you go in to the presurgery area. Who will you see? Who can go with you? Most pre-op surgery holding areas allow your family and/or friends to stay there with you until they wheel you into the surgery staging area. This is typically where they get you changed and put your IV in place, check and recheck your records, and have you visit your anesthesiologist.

Other fears may be as simple as, "Oh my gosh, I'm going to be *naked* in front of strangers!" One friend couldn't stand the thought that someone might be looking at or touching her feet while she was asleep. Another had a fear of people seeing him with a catheter bag, which is used to keep you from getting up and down for the bathroom the first day or so after the surgery. Yet another friend was concerned over people seeing her without her denture partial while in surgery. So whether your fear is having a bad hair day or a fear of not waking up, it's a real fear because it matters to you, so it goes on the list.

In reviewing this having-surgery fears column, many people find that their fears or unknowns can be crossed off or answered before they ever get to the operating room. The point of this list is that if it bothers you, it needs to be addressed.

Column 3: List Your Fears About the Potential to Fail. The third column is your fear-of-failure list. One of the biggest fears among the tens of thousands of individuals we have spoken with is that they will be the first one not to succeed at this.

- Are you afraid of missing specific foods so much that you'll eat them anyway?
- Are you afraid of damaging your pouch?
- Are you afraid of not losing any weight at all?
- Are you afraid of gaining all the weight back in six months?
- Are you afraid of not changing your eating habits?
- Do you have emotional eating issues that need to be addressed professionally via counseling?
- Are you afraid you'll feel alone?

Fear of failure comes in all forms, so don't leave anything out. Don't worry about how silly or insignificant a fear may seem. If it's enough to concern you, then it's serious enough to list and address.

Put the Columns Together to Understand Why You Will Succeed. Once you have your lists compiled, sit down and read over them. There they are, your fears, in black and white, staring up at you from those pieces of paper or from that computer screen. Putting these fears in writing gives you a much clearer picture of who you need to speak with for information and answers.

Once you know who to talk to, then it's a matter of asking questions, of however many people it takes or however many times you have to ask until you are comfortable with the answers. If you never get comfortable with the answers, then you've made your choice not to have the surgery. But if you are comfortable with the answers, then you will start to cross your fears off the lists in each column, and you may find yourself ready to go ahead with it.

By listing—and then addressing—your fears, you'll begin to see why you'll succeed at weight-loss surgery and the new way of life that comes after it. After listing all your fears, use the journal pages at the back of the book to list the reasons why you will succeed!

3

Sharing Your Decision to Have Weight-Loss Surgery

We all have friends and family members we look to for reassurance and to be there for us, and it's no different when making a decision as big as having weight-loss surgery. Dan and I know of and admire plenty of family members and friends who have cared so much about their loved ones that they, too, learned about the weight-loss surgery process, found out what to do and how to help, and got information about what to expect along the way. What a great way this is to start the process, to have your own personal support group right there with you, along with your patient support group(s)!

It's important to know, however, that not all of your friends and family are going to jump on the support bandwagon immediately. It's OK if they don't. But if their views differ drastically from yours, don't let them get you down. Arm yourself with information and share that with them. Most people who take a negative view of weight-loss surgery really don't understand the process and may not have a clue about how it will change your life. It's not necessarily that they're trying to be negative; more often, their attitude stems from fear that comes from a lack of knowledge about this procedure.

In this chapter, I'll help you prepare to face family members and friends who may be stuck in attitudes about obesity and weight loss that could make them unhelpful partners in this great life change you're making. I'll also discuss your options regarding how to communicate your surgery plans, from telling everyone right away to picking a few key supporters or even to keeping it to yourself. (Although the last option isn't common, one patient told her entire family that she was having gall bladder surgery, just to avoid potential criticism, and found her support from people other than family members.) This chapter helps you decide whom—and how much—to tell.

Finally, I'll give you practical advice and examples from our support groups for following through on whichever decision is right for you. Your own attitude and outlook are important to your success, but having support around you is also key. To make positive changes in your life, you need to surround yourself with encouraging, supportive people. This chapter gives you ideas on how to make that happen!

Finding Your Voice

If you've made the decision to have weight-loss surgery, you have to decide whether to tell people about it. Some people consider keeping the decision to themselves, for fear of having yet another weight-loss failure. They believe they would, once again, face the disappointment of well-meaning friends and family members.

These are the people who have watched you struggle with one diet after another. They cheer you on when you lose the pounds. At times, they chide you when you regain them. They may also offer tidbits of advice such as "You would be so pretty if you just lost weight," or "You really need to get your weight in check." Those comments do more damage than a physical punch, and they create scars that will be there well after the weight has disappeared. So it's no wonder we may be scared stiff that family and friends are going to judge us. This doesn't mean they *will* judge us, but it doesn't hurt to be prepared when someone brings up a question or comment you may not expect.

If you are like many of the morbidly obese, after years of feeling invisible, you may lose your voice. You may become terribly afraid of the jabs and stabs and stares and comments, and, little by little, your confidence gets eaten away, you allow these things to eat away at you until you feel almost invisible or muted. The thought of putting yourself out there, intentionally, by telling the news of your upcoming surgery scares you beyond belief.

But remember this: you are *not* invisible and you *do* have a voice. You—and you alone—get to decide about this surgery, your weight, and your life. Your self-worth is not gauged by a scale or a tape measure or the size on an article of clothing. Even though you have likely had weight-loss failures in the past—and may have felt as though you let yourself down—none of that matters today. The past is the past, and you have a fresh canvas in front of you. What are you going to choose to paint on it?

How can you find your voice and feel comfortable with this procedure? Here are a few tips:

- Your self-worth is *not* gauged by a scale or a tape measure.
- You *do* have the right to speak up for yourself and to be heard.

- You *do* have a purpose and a place in society.
- You *are* acceptable and beautiful or handsome just as you are.
- Your opinions and contributions *do* count.
- You *don't* have to be silenced by others.

For Dan and me, telling people about our weight-loss surgery has become an everyday thing. I don't mean in a mundane, ho-hum, boring, everyday kind of way. I mean a "shout-it-from-rooftops, I'm going to be healthy, I'm worth saving" excitement that swells and swells. There isn't a day that has gone by since we decided to have the surgery that we haven't talked with anyone and everyone who will listen about this procedure and how it changed our lives.

Have you ever felt so passionate about something, so deeply compelled and moved by something, that you just felt you had to let it out? You *had* to share it? Have you ever had something affect your life in such a profound way that you wanted others to experience it and feel as alive as you do now? That's the way this is for us. It's a happiness and an excitement and an exhilaration and zest for life again that is almost unexplainable.

There isn't a place Dan and I go that we don't carry before and after photos. And we're very free with passing them around and even sharing our "before" weight. Before surgery, I couldn't have ever imagined telling even the people close to me how much I weighed, much less telling stranger after stranger. At some point in the process, this number, that horrible, huge number that haunted me from my scale became a badge of honor, along with those "before" photos. No more am I ashamed of me or of my weight and size. We proudly tell everyone within earshot that at one point Dan used to weigh 400 pounds and wore a size 54 or that I weighed 264 pounds and wore a size 24.

This surgery—this tool—will help you achieve your weight-loss goals. You *will* succeed. And when you do, you will get your voice back. You're going to uncover layer after layer of emotions, feelings, desires, and objectives that you had buried—they're going to come bubbling to the surface as you begin experiencing life again.

Fighting the Myth That "You Just Have to Diet"

When we discussed having weight-loss surgery with Dan's dad, he told us that weight-loss surgery wasn't necessary. All Dan needed to do, he said, was "push away from the table." Dan was so hurt by his father's comments. We knew, of course, that what his father said didn't make practical sense; if it were that simple, there would be no need for diets or weight-loss surgery. According to the Centers for Disease Control, an estimated 65 percent of the U.S. population is overweight, with approximately 130 million individuals fighting the same battle. If it were as simple as pushing away from a table there would be no obesity and no multibillion-dollar diet industry. (The diet industry is projected to make in excess of $46 billion dollars off of diet products in the coming year.)

As Dr. Mary Vernon, a trustee of the American Society of Bariatric Physicians, explained in an interview with the Associated Press, the typical morbidly obese person she sees has already "tried mightily" to lose weight. The challenge "is giving them enough hope that it's worth trying again." The morbidly obese are typically the opposite of lazy: they're worn out, physically and spiritually, from working so hard to change.

As former members of the obese population, Dan and I worked through the entire weight-loss who's who list, trying what seemed like every plan out there: Jenny Craig, Nutrisystem, Weight Watchers, Atkins, South Beach, MediFast, Optifast, Slimfast, Carbohydrate Addicts, the Zone, and the Warrior Diet. I even took fen-phen for six straight years (it's a wonder I'm still alive). We ate cabbage soup, took over-the-counter products, and did low-fat, low-carb, liquid, boxed, bland, and dozens of other diets. Like so many other people, we kept looking for that one diet that was going to be the magic one to solve all of our weight problems.

Diets Don't Work

With all those diets, didn't we lose any weight at all? Oh yes, we lost weight. That's a part of the weight game. You realize in your twenties that you don't weigh what you used to, and you start the dieting. You lose 10 pounds, then gain 15. Then you get married. Oops, that's another 15 pounds. You diet, diet, and diet some more. You lose the 15 pounds, but eventually it comes back as 20. Then comes pregnancy. Not only does it mean you gain baby weight, but your partner gains right along with you. Then the baby comes along, and now you're eating kid snacks just because they're in front of you, and you're so tired you can't even think of going to Pilates anymore. No sleep, overwork, long days, and you forget what it's like to take care of yourself. More gaining. More dieting.

Through it all, you get more isolated. Every activity you give up, every place and person you avoid leaves you feeling more and more alone. Dan and I at least had each other, but we were cooped up and isolated from the world. And what do you do when you're indoors and you don't want to exert yourself, but you'd still like some pleasure and a feeling of company and comfort? Eat, of course.

Little did we realize that the yo-yo dieting would set up a vicious cycle that was almost impossible to change. That repeated loss of 20 pounds or 30 pounds would come back as 40 pounds, time and time again. With each cycle, we slowed our metabolisms down more and more. Lose and gain, lose and gain. Each time our metabolisms slowed, the losing got harder and the gaining got easier. Instead of solving the problem, we were making it worse.

Not all diets are inherently bad. The problem is being on a diet at all. For a diet to work, it has to be a lifestyle, for a lifetime. Most people can stick to a plan for a short time, but then they revert to old habits. There is no magic pill or magic diet or quick fix.

Hyperefficiency in Retaining Calories

Scientists now know that some bodies are just better at storing the energy from the food they eat and are hyperefficient at retaining calories. This was an advantage in famine times; if you're starving, it's good to hold onto every calorie you can. Even in good times, for most of human history, it was a long day's work just to get enough food to keep living. These days, of course, almost anyone can find an intersection with fast-food restaurants at all four corners, and if you have five dollars and five minutes to spend, you can get yourself a full day's worth of calories.

What does this mean for people who have hyperefficient, famine-resistant bodies? If they live in modern times, they have a genetic predisposition to become obese. This is true all over the world. Even on the continent of Africa, more affluent countries are finding that 10 to 15 percent of their citizens are morbidly obese. More and more countries such as China, England, Australia, Finland, Japan, Thailand, Malaysia, and the Philippines are reporting marked increases in obesity and, in particular, childhood obesity.

A New Tool for Losing Weight

Gastric bypass surgery is not another diet. Gastric bypass is stomach surgery, not brain surgery. Remember that this procedure is a *tool*—repeat that over and over! It is not a solution in and of itself, but a tool to help you lose the weight. Is this an easy tool? That depends. For some, like Dan and me, the transition from old habits to new ones is pretty easy. Other people have a more difficult time giving up old habits, and the surgery is more than they bargained for.

To be successful with weight-loss surgery, you need to treat it as the greatest tool you'll ever have for helping you develop a new, healthier lifestyle. I cannot stress to you enough the seriousness of making the most of this tool. I cannot stress to you enough the changes that *must* be made. I cannot stress to you enough that, given a little bit of effort on your part and a whole lot of wonderful things from this procedure, you can make this work for you for a lifetime. I'm not talking about another failed attempt and a life of more diets. I'm saying this tool has the possibility to be *it* for you—the elusive thing that is finally going to work that we've all hoped for. Sounds pretty amazing, doesn't it?

Have you ever heard the phrase, "you get what you give?" It applies here, because you are going to "get" in a big way when you "give" to yourself with this tool. You're going to get improved health and mobility. However, you *do* have to give: you have to give your mind over to the changes you need to make.

We recently talked with a patient who had had gastric bypass. At just a couple of weeks post-op, he was back to his old eating habits. Yes, he was losing weight because of the smaller portions he was eating, but he was setting himself up for disaster. He was rushing into eating certain foods and making bad choices, with no regard for that new, tiny pouch or the fact that he was still in the healing stages.

The people we talk to who start off cheating themselves are typically the ones we see later on who haven't lost all their weight and are trying to figure out why. These same individuals then try to go back to diet programs or diet pills instead of utilizing this tool the way it is intended. There's no need for such action. The tool is still there and functioning. It's the operator who is failing, not the surgery.

It's important to understand this weight-loss surgery is only a tool, but you have to commit to using it properly. You can't rely on the surgery itself to do it all for you. I get frustrated when I talk with patients who have surgery and then become discouraged because they *don't* dump or *don't* have issues with some foods. They try foods they shouldn't and make choices they know are not the right ones and then complain when they have no reaction. Why have surgery at all if you aren't willing to make the necessary changes?

I want you to succeed and avoid any of those physical or psychological pitfalls. I want you to be successful at this, happy with your choices, and living an active and healthy life. I want you to experience everything you've missed out on and having that same exuberance for life that we have. I want you to feel good about yourself and about taking back control over your life. And that means utilizing the tool properly and making the changes you need to make.

Answering Questions About the Safety of the Procedure

When I told my parents that Dan and I were going to have weight-loss surgery, I didn't know how they would react. Here's what they said: "You could *die*. You and Dan are going to risk dying from this! We just know it."

This kind of response is, unfortunately, very common. But how did they "just know"? They didn't. Friends and family *don't* know, either about what you're going through at your present weight or about the surgery. Even your most well-meaning supporters are likely to respond out of fear and other strong emotions.

It's understandable, of course, that your family and friends would feel concern when you go into the hospital. Up to a point, that is a good thing. But weight-loss surgery is not like other surgeries: in most cases, not having the surgery—that is, not doing anything about morbid obesity—is a walking death sentence in itself. In addition, the stomach of a morbidly obese person is not diseased, so no matter how great a job your surgeon may do, the surgery is not a cure. The cure for obesity is in changing your way of looking at food and, in turn, changing your eating habits and reshaping your emotional life to change the role of food.

If you do share your decision with others, it's amazing how many "experts" on the topic begin to crawl out of the woodwork. It seems like everyone knows someone who knew someone who talked to someone who had complications or died. If you ask for specifics (names, dates, places), you'll usually see some very rapid backpedaling—rarely, if ever, can they produce facts to back up their horror story.

Dan and I talk (either by phone, in person, or by e-mail) with thousands upon thousands of weight-loss surgery patients and people who are considering the surgery each and every month, and we've done this for years. Out of all those people, we haven't personally known a single person who has died as a result of the surgery. I'm not saying it hasn't happened, because of course it has. But statistics are overwhelmingly in favor of safety, and this is the kind of information you need to have to deflect comments from people who present you with the worst-case scenario.

Any surgery has risks, and this surgery is no exception. Don't go into major surgery without thoroughly researching the procedure, the surgeon, and the facility. This shouldn't be a spur-of-the-moment decision in any form or fashion.

Responding to the Naysayers

Naysayers, who disagree with your decision to have weight-loss surgery for whatever reason, may make it difficult for you to open up and share this important journey with others. If you experience naysayers, try, in a very kind manner, to turn the tables on them. If they tell you that you shouldn't have surgery, ask why—and ask for specifics. If they "know" someone or "read" something or "saw" something, ask from whom they heard it, where they read it, or where they saw it. By the time you have this surgery, you will have spent hours and hours, sometimes months or years, researching this procedure, and you should have the statistics to back up your decision.

Another strategy is that when those individuals start the negative talk, invite them to join you at your local support group or your online support group or message board. Once those family members and friends join in, they get a different perspective on the entire procedure. They begin to see your pain and anguish, and they see and hear, firsthand, what it's really like and what to expect in all reality. Giving them this important role not only benefits you, but it also educates them. You see, ignorance, plain old lack of knowledge about the procedure, is usually the biggest factor in their opinion. Once they get a close-up and personal view of gastric bypass surgery, the majority of those individuals will come around to understand you even better, and they may learn something about themselves along the way as well.

Don't sell yourself short. If your friends and family love you enough to be concerned for you, they can love you enough to be open-minded and support you—or at least stand alongside you.

Dealing with a Reluctant Spouse or Partner

Some people suspect that their partners won't be able to deal with the new person they're going to become. If this will be an issue with your spouse or partner, you need to address this issue head-on, and the sooner, the better. If your relationship isn't strong to begin with, and now the glue that was holding you together is going to melt away, you've got to deal with it before you have the surgery.

Communication is the key. Find out what your partner fears, what anxieties he or she has regarding this procedure. Does your partner have specific questions? Would he or she consider going with you to a support group to learn more about what to expect? As I said before, a lot of times it's just plain old fear of the unknown that causes the partner's apprehension.

Only you know how strong or weak your relationship is. Chances are, your weight has been a big part of your life together—whether you actually discuss it or not—and if your new weight is going to substantially change the dynamic of your relationship, you want to address that as soon as possible. There is more to it than just weight, and the issue is not going to go away on its own, surgery or no surgery.

I vividly recall Paloma, for example, who e-mailed Dan and me. She had waited several months before telling her husband she was considering weight-loss surgery, and, by the time she wrote to us, she was already well into the steps (testing, appointments, seminar, and so on). When she finally did tell him, he not only wasn't supportive, but he became demeaning and distant and wouldn't even discuss it with her. It turns out her husband was very insecure and felt he could "keep" her as long as she was morbidly obese and lacking in self-confidence. He felt threatened that she had stepped out of her usual complacent role and was making this decision about herself and for herself. She felt, of course, that she was doing this for them both. She wanted to be a healthier, happier, more active, and more vibrant wife. They each were looking at the same picture but seeing two very different images.

While this couple got on this rocky ground, they did opt to go into counseling. Not only did this make them closer and stronger, but it also helped them both work out emotional issues that were tying into their eating. This story was a happy ending. But they all aren't so happy. If you experience any reluctance, pushback, anger, or other strong reactions on the part of your spouse or other partner, opt for counseling. There's no shame in seeking help. Counseling is an investment in you, and you are worth the investment.

Keep in mind that, in spite of the fears of the nonsurgery spouse, amazing and positive changes can take place in your marriage or relationship after the weight loss. When Dan and I tell people that we got rid of the other couple who was sleeping with us, we first get an odd, blank stare. Then it turns to a look of shock (because for a split second they think there really was another couple in our bed). Then the realization sets in that we're talking about the 300 pounds we lost, which equals a grown man and a grown woman. Have you ever tried hugging your spouse with two people between you? That's a little far to reach. Now imagine how much more intimate you can be when all that weight is gone. There's a newfound level of intimacy that comes from within when you start to gain your self-confidence back.

When Not to Tell

There are going to be some situations where you're just not up for the confrontation—or, in some cases, the criticism—from friends, family members, or coworkers. Occasionally, individuals in our support group decide not to tell anyone. Some, as they're in the early stages, even hide their research from spouses

——————— MAKING THE CONNECTION ———————

Trish's Story: I'm about five months post-op from my weight-loss surgery, and it has made a big difference in my marriage. I had the surgery while my husband, Kurt, was on duty in Korea, so he wasn't home to see the changes I was going through every day and week. When Kurt left for Korea in July, I weighed 240 pounds and was a size 24 or 26, my heaviest weight and biggest size ever. In December, Kurt came home on a midtour Christmas visit, and I weighed 166 pounds. I was down to a size 14, which was the smallest he had ever seen me (I wore a size 18 when we met)! To this day, I'll never forget the look on his face as he walked down the terminal runway and saw me. As we walked together, he would walk ahead, look back, and say, "Wow, honey—you look good!" I think he said that three times that night! This was the ultimate good feeling—to stand proudly beside him and look good inside and out! I have 25 more pounds to go before I'll reach my goal. I can't wait until he gets off the plane again and can say, "Wow, honey" again!

or significant others. Others realize that their workplace is such a rumor mill that it's just not worth the energy of discussing the surgery and explaining it to all of their coworkers. Only you can determine when, how, or even if someone has earned the right to know.

If sharing the news is going to put you in an awkward or difficult situation, then don't do it. It's your comfort zone, and you'll know when the timing is right for you. This decision isn't about anyone else. It's about you and your health and what you determine to be best for you. You'll know when it's right for you to tell and with whom you want to discuss it. For some, telling is part of their own motivation. Others may think of telling in the same way they have discussed diets in the past: they have put themselves out there before, exposed their desires and attempts, only to fail.

It's important to keep in mind that weight-loss surgery is different from a diet. After all, have you ever seen anyone excited about going on a diet? No! But look around at the weight-loss surgery community. You'll find an entire group of people excited about this tool, the changes it offers, and the results they know are waiting.

Preparing for the Big Day

Before surgery, your range of emotions may run from excitement and nervousness to fear or even panic that something could go wrong. Some people scare themselves into skipping their surgeries. Others panic afterward, racing to the emergency room at the slightest irregularity when they could be relaxing and recuperating at home. These reactions stem from a lack of information. What you need to remember is that weight-loss surgery is a well-established, safe procedure with surprisingly little pain and a very high success rate.

Each surgeon has a program for his or her patients, which may include sample eating plans, vitamin and supplement suggestions and dosages, lab work schedules, nutritional and/or psychological preparedness classes, after-care schedules, and more. Your surgeon's program, however, may not adequately prepare you for all the concerns you may have about the big day. In this chapter, I talk about what you can do before your surgery to help you have a positive experience with the least amount of stress.

Recognizing That Support Groups Are Your Safety Net

Dan and I like to think of the following mnemonic, which spells out "support," when describing what a support group can offer or be:

Sharing
Uplifting
Peer support
Positive
Open and honest
Reality check
Thought-provoking

In the following sections, I help you understand the benefits of joining a support group now—*before* your surgery! I also help you find the local or online group that's best for you.

———————— MAKING THE CONNECTION ————————

Joni's Story: I was always the chubby one. In elementary school, I was the little fat kid who wanted so bad to fit in, to be able to play dodgeball and not be the target all the time, or to play kickball and be able to run as fast as the rest of the kids. In high school, I got by being the class cut-up and actually making fun of myself to fit in. I had girlfriends to hang with but, then again, I had a car. My father died while I was in high school of a massive heart attack. To compensate for the loss, I ate.

As an adult, it moved from my own school experiences to ones with my children. They never condemned me for my weight or even seemed to notice. But my heart would sink when there were school functions for parents to attend and I could barely fit in the seats or would get winded just walking to the classroom. Diet after diet, I tried them all. Oh, I lost weight, and I then gained twice as much when I stopped the diet programs.

It's funny what can finally trigger your decisions for surgery. I am an Emergency Medical Technician, and once I was told by my boss that I would have to start looking "more professional" by tucking in my shirt. So I would "tuck" my shirt in by just folding it under and making it appear to be tucked in. This was actually the turning point for me. I was tired of looking sloppy, not only at work but at home, and I was tired of the stares, giggles, comments, and constant ridicule.

Several people I know had undergone gastric bypass surgery, and their results were amazing. I joined an online support group prior to the surgery, and I found the best one on the Net. We are a family, and I have been dubbed "the Queen Worrywart" of the board.

On my surgery day, I walked into the hospital a morbidly obese woman for the last time. This surgery would change my life. Since the surgery, I have lost 122 pounds. I have flown in an airplane and traveled to places I have never seen. I have met some new and terrific friends through our online support group. But the best part of having this surgery is knowing I can now enjoy every minute of my grandchildren. I can get on the floor with them, I can run outside with them, and I can hold them closer than I could have ever held them without the surgery.

This surgery has changed my life, for the better. Today, I do tuck my shirt in and stand proud; I am as professional looking now as my colleagues. Better than that, I feel good, and my friends and family are proud of me. So am I.

Understanding the Benefits of
Joining a Support Group

Many people find that a support group becomes like a second family. Whether you join a local group, an online group, or both, the members of your support group are people you can truly rely on. In these groups, weight-loss surgery patients (and patients-to-be) share every possible detail and discuss every topic. Some discussions may be more pleasant than others, but nothing is off limits. Every time someone posts what they think is a "dumb" question on our website, the Weight Loss Surgery Connection (thewlsconnection.com), others will say they were wondering the exact same thing! You're not alone—not in your thoughts, your fears, or your experiences. And getting that support from others is the primary benefit of joining a support group.

Nowhere is the camaraderie more apparent than at a support group meeting. You'll have an entire community that understands what it's like to try dieting and fail, what it's like to jump through the insurance company hoops, and what you can expect in the coming days or months. You can discuss whatever your heart desires, knowing the feedback you get comes from a genuine place of caring and empathy. You'll feel their concern and compassion, and you'll find yourself feeling the same way about others in your group as well.

Maybe you've had a bad day and just need someone there to listen. There are others who are ready to lend an ear. No matter what time of the day or night (especially if you're online), there's someone else right there with you. Whether you're laughing, crying, rejoicing, or just looking to chat, there's always someone to connect with. A support group truly is an extended family.

To gain the full benefit of being a part of the group, however, it's important to be brutally honest. That's not to say that your comments should ever be nasty, because there's always a polite way to say things. The care and concern behind every comment should always be evident. But honesty and accountability are essential for making a support group work. Who better than your peers—people who have walked in your shoes—to call you on the carpet if they see you heading down a path paved with poor choices? Most group members are looking for that honesty and accountability to help them stay the course.

Joining a Support Group *Before* the Surgery

If you'd looked in on Dan and me as we prepared for our surgery, you might not have thought we would succeed in the long term. We had no outside support, no community, no message boards, no other resources. Our parents and other family members did not understand our choice. We had become badly isolated, and the two of us felt cut off from the rest of the world. And yet we found the support we needed in each other, bouncing questions off each other, reviewing research together, talking it all through, and going through the procedure together. Throughout that process, we reinforced our confidence that weight-loss surgery was the right choice for us.

Most people don't have a built-in weight-loss partner sitting in the next room, which is why we actively support other weight-loss surgery patients today. After our surgeries, we wanted to offer our knowledge and support to others so they could share our experiences and the experiences of many of the thousands of successful weight-loss patients we talk with on a regular basis.

Getting support is not an extra nicety that helps with this "real thing," the surgery. Instead, the emotional changes in your life and the shift in your habits are "the real thing." A support group helps you get to that new place in your life. And well after your surgery, even when you've reached your goal weight and are in your maintenance phase, you'll find that support is even more important. (See Chapter 8 for more on long-term support after your surgery.)

It's important to join a support group before surgery. In this "before" stage, you'll be accepted by a family of supporters. You can be comfortable talking about and exploring how you became morbidly obese. It's about getting acceptance for who you are, no matter what your size, and finding the support foundation to help you through this process.

No one wants to undertake something as extreme as weight-loss surgery all alone. We don't know if weight-loss surgery is right for you, but we know how much it can help to have others to talk to—and maybe even confide in—while you learn about your choices and make your decision. If you choose to have the surgery, we know how precious it is to have someone with you every step of the way, helping you succeed and giving you the kind of postoperative family of support that can make your dreams of a new life come true.

Don't wait until you're suffering to find the support you need. Although there is never a bad time to join a support group, the best time to join is *before* you have surgery. You need to hear other people's stories for yourself to prepare for the procedure, the recovery, and the changes in eating immediately afterward. A few doses of vivid storytelling by people who have already undergone the surgery will prepare you for what to expect and ease your mind when going into your own surgery.

Group support is a great comfort before surgery and provides an invaluable service that will carry you through a lifetime. Support is there any hour, any day, whenever you need that connection. Having the right group of people to support you is as important as having the right surgeon operate on you. Talking with your peers and sharing fears, milestones, new information, and suggestions will become a lifeline that you can rely on.

Finding the Right Support Group

Support groups are usually either local, in which you meet with people in your geographic area, or online, where you meet "virtually" via the Internet. You can find a local support group by asking your surgeon or bariatric center or checking with your hospital. You can find online groups by searching the Internet or going to established sites such as thewlsconnection.com, http://groups.msn.com/gastricbypasssupport, or obesityhelp.com.

If there's a local group affiliated with your own surgical practice, consider joining it, because it will provide a place for consistent information, using the same guidelines. There's nothing wrong, however, with joining a program that isn't affiliated with your own surgeon. In fact, some people find they like these other programs better. Just keep in mind that no one program is going to be perfect or have all the answers to suit everyone. Keep looking until you find the one that fits you best. In fact, find several. No one says you have to belong to only one group. The more support and the broader range of information you're exposed to, the better.

Local Support Groups. With a local group, you have everything you need right in front of you. If the group is organized through your surgeon's practice, you will have other people who can share their firsthand experience of surgery and recovery. They can walk you through what to expect at your local hospital, because they've been there, with the same doctors and nurses you'll be working with. These people may be the very best source of support for you, as their experience will likely be very similar to yours. And having success stories right before your very eyes is a comfort in itself.

When you're with your local group, spend time asking them lots of questions. Start off with your checklist of questions, recognizing that, as you hear more shared stories, your list of questions will multiply. Listen closely to the stories, and catch all the details from each level of experience. Together, the members of your local group are like a treasure chest filled with gems of information that you will accumulate just from being there and participating.

Some people find they are shy when it comes to face-to-face groups. They'll go and listen, but they won't truly speak up and join in. That's OK, too. While active participation at meetings is certainly beneficial, it is not a requirement. Even if you don't speak up, you'll likely find friends galore who understand exactly what you're feeling. If you feel too shy to join in but you have a lot of questions to ask, an online group (discussed in the following section) might be the right supplement to an in-person group.

Online Support Groups. Some people find an online group to be an easier format for them to step out and ask questions without feeling self-conscious, as may be the case in a room filled with people. Perhaps it is easier to be brutally honest (although never rude or tactless!) and vent all your questions and concerns online. The message board format also gives you the opportunity just to lurk, which means reading others' posts without posting anything yourself. Another advantage of an online support group is that it affords you the luxury of thinking through what you want to say and editing it before posting. Finally—and

─────────────── MAKING THE CONNECTION ───────────────

Faye's Story: At age 56, I knew I had to do something about my weight. Thanks to diet pills (amphetamines) that were easy to get, I weighed 119 pounds when I got married in 1970. A year later, though, I had gained 60 pounds, and then with each pregnancy, I gained 60 to 80 more. I could lose weight with diet pills, but it never lasted.

Over the next 30 years, I tried every diet imaginable and had so many exercise books and videos and so much equipment that I could have opened my own store. I spent thousands of dollars—almost $12,000 since 2002 when I started tracking—to lose weight! I was hypnotized, was wrapped in Saran Wrap for three months, bought patches, joined Weight Watchers, tried Atkins and the South Beach diet, did Fit for Life, ate the cabbage soup diet, and went on the grapefruit diet. Nothing worked long term.

Meanwhile, I was on antidepressants, had joint issues, and was diagnosed with fibromyalgia. My physician recommended weight-loss surgery, and I found the process pretty simple. First, there was six months of weight management and getting everything submitted to the insurance company. But once it was submitted, I was approved in a week.

I then joined the online MSN Gastric ByPass Support Group and read, read, read! I found the information to be so honest and helpful—I knew exactly what to expect, what to do, and what not to do. Every question was answered, and questions I'd never even thought about were answered. I felt confident and ready for my life-changing event, thanks to my support group.

The thought of living on liquids for two weeks prior to surgery was the most daunting, but with the help of my support group, I did it: the day I started the liquid diet, I weighed 232.5; the morning of surgery, I was down to 214.

I am now almost six months post-op and have lost almost 70 pounds and 42 inches. Walking is no longer a chore, and I can fasten the seat belt on the plane with room to spare. I now love to shop, and my husband is looking forward to shopping at Victoria's Secret for me! I have no idea what weight or size I want to be. I just know, deep in my soul, that when I'm where I need to be, I'll know. Weight-loss surgery may not be for everyone, but for me, it was the right decision. With family, friends, and my online support family, I know I'll succeed!

perhaps the greatest benefit—is that, online, you can get the support you need right when you need it, not just during a weekly or monthly meeting.

No matter what phase you are in, you can get benefits from this tool. If you're pre-op, you can get encouraged and excited by reading others' success stories. You may be in contact with someone who is having surgery just a week or two before your own schedule. Or there may be people who are a month, two months, a year, or even two years post-op, and you can get enthused by reading their accounts, knowing this is what you have to look forward to.

Inviting Friends and Family to Your Presurgery Support-Group Meetings

If you want to feel even closer to your support group, you might want to think about inviting friends and family members to join as well. They're welcome to ask questions and interact with the group. After all, the more support you have before the surgery and throughout your recovery and weight loss, the better your chances for long-term success. Also, the more your family and friends understand this procedure and the obstacles you'll encounter with each stage, the better prepared they will be to give you extra backing. Asking family and friends to join you in your support group also includes them in something that you have deemed as essential to getting your life back. Your friends and family are a part of that life, and they will want to do anything and everything they can to make your journey a positive one.

Clearing Your Schedule

Only you and your surgeon know what kind of timeline you'll need for your surgical experience. Depending on the procedure you opt for, your own physical condition, and the surgeon's skill level, the surgery itself can be very quick or can be extensive. Some surgeons perform laparoscopic Roux-en-Y (see Chapter 2) in as little as 30 minutes, but others need to take hours on end due to unforeseen issues such as hernias or old scar tissue. Talk with your surgeon about his or her typical surgical times.

The amount of time you are hospitalized varies as well. Most weight-loss surgical procedures call for at least a one-night hospital stay, followed by recuperation at home. But some people have to stay longer.

One frequently asked question is, "How soon can I go back to work?" The answer depends on your recovery. On average, patients return to work within two weeks; others take the maximum amount of time allowed off by their employers, whether that's more or less than two weeks. The typical patient is up and walking soon after surgery; in fact, the more you get moving, the quicker you'll feel better and be ready to go out in the world again.

Making Your Kitchen Healthy

The waiting weeks, between insurance approval and surgery, is the perfect time to go through your pantry, refrigerator, and cabinets and clear out the things you don't want or need around the house. You can then replace those foods with the foods you will need after your surgery. The two following sections tell you what to throw away and what to stock up on.

Knowing What to Throw Away

It's time to clean out all the junk in your kitchen once and for all, removing all sugars and sugary foods, all high-carb foods, and anything else with low nutritional value. Clean out your pantry and refrigerator, and restock both with healthier choices. If you're unsure whether an item is healthy, read the label, checking the carbohydrates, protein, and sugars. If you're honest with yourself, you know what's in your individual pantry or refrigerator, and you know what's healthy and what isn't. It's time to do a good clean-out and rid yourself of those old snacks or empty-nutritional-value choices. A partial list of things to get rid of includes:

Cookies
Chips
Pretzels
Waffles
Pancake mix
Ice cream
Doughnuts
Candy bars
White flour
Pasta
Rice
Cereals
Carbonated beverages

Reality check: you are going to have to be vigilant from now on to make sure that these unhealthy foods stay out of the house. It doesn't take much for old habits to creep back in and take over; sometimes just the sight of doughnuts in your pantry, where they used to always reside, can be enough to throw you off your good intentions. Remember, you are in control and these are *your* choices. These steps are all for your recovery and long-term success.

Stocking Up on the Right Stuff

Once you've done your kitchen clean-out, then it's time to stock up on the things you do need. Before weight-loss surgery, it is important to prepare your family for the changes they'll be seeing in the kitchen. Not only are you going to be eating healthier, but this is the perfect opportunity to ensure that your family eats better as well. Right after the surgery, your momentum and support will run high, so it's a great time to give everyone a fresh start.

You are the focus here, of course, so the advice in this section pertains specifically to you.

Measuring Devices and Other Tools. For starters, you want to be sure you have containers that help you determine exactly how much you're eating. You can't assume portion size; you have to measure, measure, measure! One of the most common pitfalls I see is people thinking they are eating 2 ounces when they're actually eating 8 ounces—and then they can't understand why they feel poorly after eating. Well, they're overeating! In addition, smaller dishes will match your smaller portion sizes and not make your servings seem so small! Here are some ideas:

- **Measuring cups and spoons.** Buy yourself a good set of small measuring cups and spoons. Shot glasses can be quite helpful, too, when it comes to measuring. Look especially for a 4-ounce measuring cup for your 2-ounce portions— the portion won't look too tiny, but you also won't spill and make a mess.
- **Food scale.** You can find these at kitchen stores or mass merchandisers; they usually run $3 to $20. Scales are a great way to determine exactly how much you're eating.

- **Smaller dishes.** A great big soup bowl is going to look pretty overwhelming when you put your 2 ounces of soup in it. Ramekins (custard cups) make a great soup bowl for small portions. Salad plates make nice dinner plates. Ice cube trays are perfect for freezing small portions of broth or soup. Very small food storage containers, too, are great for storing and freezing portions.
- **Smaller utensils.** Many people opt for baby or toddler utensils in the beginning to acclimate themselves to eating smaller bites and taking smaller sips.
- **Slow cooker.** Look into buying a slow cooker, if you don't already have one. When you're making broths and soups for the first few weeks of your postsurgery eating plan, a slow cooker can be a real lifesaver. It will be a kitchen staple for you in the future, too.

Good Foods. Although your surgeon may prescribe one of a wide range of eating plans, the consistent part of any of these plans is easing foods back in. Slow and steady. That new stomach of yours needs time to heal. There will be plenty of time to add in textures in just a few short weeks, so don't rush! You didn't get to this stage overnight, and the biggest favor you can do for yourself is to make the most of the early weeks after weight-loss surgery. Chapter 5 gives you the specific details on how to eat during your postoperative period, but you do want to start stocking up well before your big day.

Here's a list of what to stock up on:

Water
Soups (homemade, from a local restaurant, or canned)
Sugar-free Jell-O
100 percent fruit juices (no sugar added)

Frozen 100 percent whole fruit bars (no sugar added)
Variety of herbs and spices

Soup is an excellent postsurgery food, as long as it's not high in sodium. Consider making the soups yourself so you can control what goes into them. Even if you're not much of a cook, you can make the simple recipes in Appendix A. When Dan and I were preparing for our surgeries, I cooked a batch of chicken soup and a batch of beef soup and froze them in ice cube trays; then I transferred the cubes into freezer bags or freezer containers. Each cube was one ounce, so it was easy transfer this frozen soup from the freezer to a small dish and into the microwave. It also made it easy for us to keep track of measurements and have quick preparation at mealtimes.

Another option is to talk with your favorite restaurant about their soups. If the restaurant is one you know well and trust, you may find the chefs there to be very accommodating. You can purchase fresh soups and freeze them or just have them on hand when the time comes.

If you go with canned soups, please start reading the labels. Many canned soups are very high in sodium, which you want to steer clear of.

Herbs and spices are on the list because your tastes will likely change such that even the simplest things, like water, may take on a whole new dimension. I can now taste every mineral in different waters, and that's not unusual. Many people find, over time, that they can drink only specific brands of water or water with flavors added. With that in mind, you'll want to pick up a variety of bottled waters to choose from.

Just because you are on liquids or purees in those early weeks doesn't mean that they have to taste bland. Once my husband and I were allowed to move onto cream soups and purees, we added vegetable juices. One of our favorite additions was a spicy Bloody Mary mix. We began experimenting with a variety of herbs and spices in our soups, too. Flavor will make such a difference in your satisfaction level and will help to avoid head hunger (see Chapter 7). Feed your senses while you fill your stomach so you get overall satisfaction instead of just filling a void.

Protein Supplements and Vitamins. Last, but not least, on the short list are vitamin and protein supplement samples that you may even get from your doctor. The vitamins are to ensure that you're receiving all the nutrients you need, and the protein supplements are for you to use if you're not getting enough protein from your foods.

Don't stock up too much on any one type of protein supplement or vitamin because they just might not work for you after surgery. Before buying, talk with your favorite local health food store and ask their policy. Explain to them what procedure you are having done, and you'll find most are quite helpful in obtaining a variety of samples for you. Most of the people who work at health food stores have made their living by helping people with unique food requirements! If you've never been to a health food store, look online or in your Yellow Pages under "health foods" or "natural foods."

For a helpful way to itemize what you need to buy to prepare for surgery, you can use the journal pages in Appendix B.

Packing for the Hospital

I've spent many hours talking with patients about the list of things to take—and not to take—to the hospital. Some people think they need to pack as if they were going on a long trip. In this situation, however, less is more. For that reason, I've split this section in two parts: what to take with you, and what to leave at home.

Deciding What to Take with You

You won't need much at the hospital. A list of what to bring includes:

Comfortable two-piece pajamas
Slippers or nonskid booties
Pillow
Lip balm
A book or magazine
Comfortable clothes to go home in

Definitely bring comfy pajamas. Hospital gowns can feel scratchy, and they're drafty. A pair of loose-fitting, two-piece pajamas will also be a plus with everyone who will be in and out of your room. The medical staff will be checking your vital signs and your incisions frequently; two-piece pajamas will allow them to check incisions and still give you the comfort of being covered up. You'll also be strolling down the hall a lot, and when you do, you'll be thankful that you have your pajamas on.

You don't want to forget slippers, either. Many hospitals provide booties with nonskid grips on the bottom, so ask whether your hospital or surgery center does. If not, you'll want to pack them. You don't want to be walking the halls in bare feet on cold, slick floors.

If you have a difficult time sleeping on any pillow other than your own, consider taking one of your own. Extra pillows can be requested from the nursing staff, but some people find their own pillow to be more comforting to them.

Lip balm comes in handy, because dry lips can be frustrating. If you're not allowed any liquids for the first 24 hours (and that depends on your doctor and the procedure), most hospitals will have citrus-flavored glycerin swabs available upon request for that dry mouth. Ask your doctor whether you're also allowed to use sugar-free mints to hydrate your mouth. You will certainly be advised to not chew them, though.

It also helps to pack a book or magazine if you get bored easily. Bring something comfy to wear home. And check with your surgeon, bariatric center, or hospital ahead of time to see whether they need a driver's license copy on your arrival.

Finally, remember that packing light is something you'll be thankful for when you get ready to go home. There's no need to be carrying a lot of nonessentials, especially when you remember that there's no heavy lifting after surgery. The journal pages in Appendix B include space for you to list the items you want to take the hospital.

Deciding What to Leave at Home

Leave all personal or expensive items at home. This includes jewelry, watches, purses, wallets, money, iPods, and cell phones (which are often not permitted by the hospital anyway). Unless you really need them, they'll just be a nuisance to keep track of. If you do intend to take personal items, make certain you have friends or family you can trust with your valuables. These are recommendations by the hospitals to protect you and the attendants as well.

The most important things to leave at home, though, are your old attitude and beliefs about food, because they are all about to change. You know what old bad habits got you—a trip to the hospital for surgery! Those old habits didn't do you any favors, but now you have the chance to change them all. Not only are you undergoing surgery on your stomach, you're undergoing surgery on your choices. This is your chance to cut out the negatives and replace them with the positives that are going to make you succeed in the long term. This is a time to start fresh, with a clean slate. This is the effort that's going to pay off once and for all. Your new, healthy future is waiting for you.

Tracking Your Progress on the Path to Success

After the surgery, as you begin to lose weight quickly, you need to be able to see and remember those "before" pounds, measurements, feelings, and so much more. This information is going to give you a record of your journey. It's also going to keep you motivated. As the weeks, months, and years pass, you can look at your records of your progress and see where you were and what you've gone through. It'll be a reminder of what you don't want to return to!

For this reason, it's important to start making your "before" records the week before your surgery. You can immediately begin tracking the results of your surgery when you get home and those pounds start to fall off.

For your weigh-ins and measurements, be sure to write these numbers in a log. You can design a log yourself, get one from your surgeon, or buy one at a stationery store. It can be as simple as handwritten notes. If you prefer to organize your measurements on your computer, there are a lot of great software programs designed specifically for tracking weight loss and measurements. Some are even accessible via PDA, desktop, or both. It's not necessary to get a specific program—you can set up your own formatting in a Word document or a spreadsheet if you don't wish to pay for a software program. What is important is to find the log that works best for you, one that you'll use regularly.

Taking "Before" Pictures of Your Body

To begin your record keeping, it is best to start with the one thing you probably hate the most: the camera. Yes, I mean pictures, pictures, and more pictures! During the week before your surgery, have someone you trust take pictures of your body from every angle. Find a blank wall and put on clothing that is going to show your true size, something fitted. You're going to be taking progress photos regularly until you reach your goal weight, and you'll want to use the same location for the sake of consistency. Many people dress in clothing that will be easy to replicate during the course of their weight loss (bathing suit, sports bra and shorts, T-shirt and shorts, and so on) to better emphasize the changes. Take photos of your full front, back, and both sides, and remember to photograph from the same distance for consistency.

You may also want to go through your old photos and pull out some pictures of you at your largest to keep with your records. I know it's painful, but consider this the starting point of your healing. This will be the last time you see yourself like that. And although you may not think so now, those photos will be something you actually become proud of later, a badge of honor showing where you began and what you have accomplished.

Many people regret not having those "before" photos, so make sure to take them. You may even want to keep one of them in a visible place, after you've gotten to your goal, as a daily reminder of where you never want to return.

Weighing In

The next step is weighing in right before your surgery. Believe me, I know what's it's like to truly hate that scale. But it's soon going to become one of your favorite things in the house. If you don't have a scale, be sure to purchase one before the surgery. Record your weight (yes, in writing, in your log!) either the night before or the morning of your surgery. After you get home, you'll want to use this same scale to begin weighing in regularly.

Morning is the best time to weigh in. As soon as you rise, step on the scale—before breakfast, with your clothes off. Doing this first thing in the morning will give you the truest picture of your weight (and, therefore, of your weight loss) because everything you eat or drink, everything you wear, and every activity you do can affect your weight one way or the other. Normal body fluctuations are to be expected, especially in women, but morning weigh-ins will give you the truest assessment of your progress.

Taking Your Measurements

After you've collected the pictures and weighed in, now comes another "fun" activity, taking your measurements. Make a list of measurement areas from head to toe in your log. You will be amazed at what will change in the next few months. From the largest areas, stomach and hips, to the smallest areas, wrists and ankles, you are going to see dramatic changes over your entire body.

Here are the measurements you want to take:

Neck
Chest
Bust
Waist
Hips
Abdomen
Thighs (both)
Calves (both)
Ankles (both)
Upper arms (both)
Lower arms (both)
Wrists (both)

A sample recording sheet is available in the journal pages in Appendix B. This is your accounting and accountability record in black and white. Just the act of writing these things down is important because it makes you stop and think about how far you've

————————— MAKING THE CONNECTION —————————

Noreen's Story: In 1980, my husband, Jack, and I were in a motor-cycle accident. We did not know what the effects of that one small incident would have on us for the following years. It was 10 years before there was a real clue that something was seriously wrong. I would have surgeries, mountains of prescription drugs, and count-less doctor visits. Over the next 20 years it all crept up on me, and I was in such serious pain that my life came to a halt. I was unable to do even the smallest things for myself. I couldn't even get myself to the doctor, so I had to rely on my husband (who had to miss work) or have the senior center in town give me rides to the hospital for treatment. I weighed 240 pounds and had no idea how I would ever lose any of that weight when I couldn't even walk 50 feet without getting winded.

During this time, I started looking around online for information about weight-loss surgery. I was desperate for anything that could help me gain some kind of life back. I found the Gastric Bypass Support Group at http://groups.msn.com/gastricbypasssupport. That incredible support is how I made it through the next year of my life waiting to have the surgery while I was trying to cope with lack of mobility, fibromyalgia, three bulging discs in my cervical spine, and sciatica.

I finally had my surgery and couldn't believe that within weeks after surgery, I had lost a significant amount of weight: 50 pounds, then 60, then 70, 80, 90, and it was still melting away. It was amaz-ing. My family members, who were all so afraid for me before the surgery, thought that something would go wrong. For me, even if something were to go wrong, it had to be better than what was going on before the surgery.

By the time I lost the first 40 pounds, I was feeling better than I had for years. I was getting out and even started a garden. I looked like I did when I was a teenager. Everyone was amazed at how I felt and looked. My husband was so proud of me; he even bought me a little statue of an angel that stood for courage. I was just amazed at everyone's reaction.

My sister and niece saw my results and later had weight-loss surgery as well. Now, my husband, Jack, recently had weight-loss surgery and is doing very well—another success story in the making. It is amazing how many people can be touched by what you personally accomplish, without you even knowing you are doing anything to inspire them. I am now working full-time and am off all pain medications. I have my life back and have inspired others to take their lives back. I have never felt so good about myself. I've never felt so good, period!

---

come and how much (or, eventually, how little) you have left to go. Your measurements are going to be one of your biggest encouragements, especially when you hit a plateau (see Chapter 7).

Starting a Journal

Another habit I encourage everyone on the Weight-Loss Surgery Connection to adopt before surgery is keeping a journal in addition to the weight and measurements log. How else will you remember your state of mind and your feelings at the beginning of your weight-loss journey? Most weight-loss surgery candidates have spent many years eating absentmindedly or simply going through the motions of trying to lose weight. But with a journal, as you write down everything you eat, in addition to how you're feeling, you can't help but slow down and think. You can utilize the journal pages in Appendix B to get started.

A journal is something to start not only after the surgery but before, too. Record not just what food you ate, but how much, how fast, how often, what it tasted like, how it made you feel, how long it took to feel full. Getting to know what you are eating as well as why, how much, and what it tastes like are all important bits of information that should make their way into your food journal. (See Chapter 5 for more information on keeping a journal.)

The next time you go to the grocery store, wander the aisles. Read the labels on various kinds of food and jot down what you see. What an enlightening experience this is! You'll find information you probably skipped over before. For example, you're going to get a big wake-up call when you start looking at ingredients, something you may not have done much of before. Look at the protein, carbohydrate, and sugar content, and look at serving sizes. It's kind of a pain, but the effort of putting nutritional information from food labels and all sorts of other information into your food logs is a minor concession for the payoff you'll receive.

You are going to be portion-size conscious for the rest of your life. You need to know how much nutrition various foods provide, in small portion sizes. Recognizing this information and noting it in your journal will help you develop healthy habits and choices.

For your initial entry, write about your "last supper"—that real meal you think you'll never have again after surgery. Many people splurge on the foods they think they're going to miss, but most people look back on that "last supper" and either laugh at the choices or are repulsed by them. It will help you to know that most people who work through recovery and lose the weight find they aren't missing anything at all after surgery! But until you reach that point, record that last meal in detail.

What to Expect on the Big Day

Everyone's experience of surgery is different. I'll share what Dan's and my day of surgery was like, to give you one perspective. I hope our experience will help you feel less of that fear of the unknown.

Per doctor's orders, Dan and I had no food or drink after midnight the night before surgery. The next morning we both bounced out of bed early, all ready for our big day! Your own surgery time will be set by your surgeon's staff, but our surgeries were scheduled for morning. For me, this was a big deal, because I didn't want to be waiting around all day with nothing to eat or drink. It may sound silly, but not having to go without water any longer than I had to was my only real concern.

Once we arrived at the hospital, we headed for the presurgical area to be admitted and prepped for surgery. We were allowed to have family and friends with us, and the nurses and anesthesiologist were there to comfort us and answer any and all questions. They put us in a small room where we could get changed, and then they put in our IVs and confirmed all our paperwork (verifying who we were, the procedure we were having, and so on). They also bagged up our personal belongings for transfer to our room after surgery.

Once it was time for surgery, we were wheeled into a presurgery holding area. The surgical nurses were very caring; they gave us heated blankets to keep us warm and had plenty of smiles and hand squeezes to reassure us. Between the smiles and the hand pats and all of the caring comments, we felt totally relaxed. We were in the holding area for only a short time, just long enough to reconfirm our paperwork once again.

Next, our surgeon came by to visit, and we were wheeled into the operating room. Neither Dan nor I remember much of this part at all. The next thing we knew, we were waking up in recovery and being taken to our rooms. Three hours later, we were up and walking the hallways.

When we got to see our "war wounds," we discovered we had only six tiny incisions from our laparoscopic Roux-en-Y surgery (see Chapter 2) and no visible outward stitches. We didn't even have bandages. There was a clear liquid bandage over the incisions, but no other visible signs of the procedure for us.

Our discomfort was minimal, but the nursing staff was ready to offer a painkiller pump or shots, if we so chose. After the first day, we didn't need any painkillers stronger than Tylenol. By getting up and walking around, you recover and feel better much faster than if you lie or sit.

Keep in mind that everyone's recovery is very different, but I can't tell you how many times I've heard others recount the same experience. Most are quite surprised at how simple it really is.

Preparing for Potential Side Effects

Weight-loss surgery is well established, and, generally speaking, the side effects are minimal. For example, Dan and I felt well enough to drive ourselves home from the hospital after the surgery (although not everyone will feel this good!), even stopping at the store to pick up some juice. Neither of us felt a substantial amount of pain, nothing that a little Tylenol wouldn't take care of.

The day after we returned home, we were stir-crazy and had to get out of the house. We went to the nearest major mass merchandiser just to wander around. At six days post-op, we felt good enough to go on a long bike ride—something we hadn't had the energy or inclination to do in years. What a rush it was to walk or peddle down the bike path thinking about the changes we were seeing every single day! It was the first time in dozens of years where we felt we were finally going to succeed at getting healthy and being able to maintain that healthy lifestyle.

Our surgery and post-op experiences are not unique. We know from our website and message board that the majority of people who have weight-loss surgery not only feel an exhilarating reconnection to a self that they had long forgotten, but also do not experience much post-op pain. They are capable of taking care of themselves once home and getting back to work in a short amount of time.

Although side effects are usually minimal, there are three side effects that can badly frighten patients. Unfortunately, I have been told by numerous people that their doctors failed to educate them about these potential post-op side effects, causing them unnecessary alarm when they did experience them. In this section, I help you understand the three major side effects of the surgery, so as to alleviate some of that shock and fear if these do occur.

Gas Pains

Gas pains can sometimes be so sharp that you may feel like you're having a heart attack. These pains reach much higher than you might expect, even up to your shoulders. This is a result of the air your surgeon will use to inflate your abdomen during the procedure. It's easy to imagine that any pain you might feel in your chest is a serious complication, even a heart attack, but it's usually just gas.

Getting up and walking around helps to ease the discomfort. The main reason to move around after surgery is to prevent blood clots, but it is also a huge help in moving that gas out. Within a few hours after your surgery, you'll likely be strolling through the hallways. Well, not exactly strolling—perhaps shuffling is more accurate. Hang onto that IV pole and your nurse, and then go slow and easy.

Gas pains really can be severe and can last for days. If moving around isn't alleviating all the pain, you may want to try using a pillow or a rolled-up towel to apply pressure to areas that feel bloated or painful.

———————　MAKING THE CONNECTION　———————

Peg's Story: I've been obese all my life but didn't know I was fat until first grade when the other kids let me know about it right away. I remember being on Weight Watchers the first time when I was in third grade and taking belly dance lessons with adult members of my family when I was about 10 in an effort to help me lose weight. I'd drop a few pounds, but never enough to get into the normal weight category. For a couple of months in grade school, I was even on doctor-prescribed medication to lose weight. These were diet pills—and I was only in grade school.

I couldn't even tell you what I weighed when I started high school. Luckily for me, I was at least "tolerated" well in my little high school. I had a lot of friends, both male and female, but I never had a date. Moving on to a large state university, I went from being a big fish in a little pond, to being a fat little fish in a great big pond. My sense of self-esteem plummeted as I became more and more afraid of being ignored or mistreated because of my weight, so rather than try, I just retreated into myself and avoided any kind of clubs and group activities in college.

During my adult life, I worked with some great people, and although I always had a lot of friends, I rarely went out on dates. I was always afraid of being made fun of. I found myself fighting health problems, starting with high blood pressure and osteoarthritis in my knees, and moving on to steadily worsening diabetes and severe edema in my feet, ankles, and calves. I dieted over and over again, losing maybe 30 to 50 pounds before stalling out and giving up, only to regain the amount I had lost plus another 20 or 30 pounds on top of it. All through the years, the idea of weight-loss surgery scared me to death as I had heard stories of people suffering worse health issues after the surgery or even dying.

However, the final wake-up call came when, at the age of 41, I had a doctor's visit at which my weight had reached an all-time high of 373 pounds. I was absolutely miserable. I thought about whether I wanted to live to see 60 years old and decided to seriously look into the surgery as my insurance had begun coverage of the Roux-en-Y procedure that year. I called the insurance company and found out the requirements and what doctors they covered, but it took me about a month to finally make the call to the surgery program to start the process. Once I started the process, because of my comorbidities and all my efforts to follow the pre-op procedures, I flew through the insurance-approval process and was scheduled for surgery quickly. On the day of surgery, I weighed in at 326 pounds.

Fast-forward to the current day and I now weigh 223, down 150 pounds from my highest weight. Within 10 days after surgery, my doctor took me off both of my diabetes medications. By the time I reached 260 pounds, I was also off the medications for hypertension. Although my pre-op sleep study showed I had sleep apnea, I had to go off of the CPAP machine right after surgery. I lost weight so quickly that they couldn't adjust the machine low enough for me to be able to use it, and subsequent tests showed my sleep apnea had also disappeared. My ankles are now skinny, too!

What's more, I've been dating a nice guy, whom I asked out. No more waiting around or being a wallflower for me! Besides losing the weight and regaining my health, I gained my confidence back after so many years. Life is wonderful thanks to weight-loss surgery, and I would do it again in a heartbeat.

Also keep in mind that, no matter how much your doctor dismisses gas pain, you never want to ignore pain. If something hurts, disclose it to your surgeon or a nurse immediately.

Dehydration

Another serious post-op issue is dehydration. Many weight-loss surgery patients complain of not being able to take in their liquids—at least 64 ounces per day—in the early post-op days.

When you come out of surgery, it's important to begin drinking water as soon as your doctor allows. For some that may be 24 hours after surgery; for others, it may involve slow sips the first day, which your nurse will remind you to take.

When you get home and are working on getting in your fluids, think of it on a smaller scale. Try not to feel overwhelmed when you hear a number like 64 ounces of water going in that tiny little pouch. If you break it down over a 16-hour day, 64 ounces of water means consuming several swallows every 15 to 30 minutes. That's only a few tablespoons at a time. Use a timer or your cell phone alarm to remind you. Sipping water often is a habit you want to develop right after the surgery, one that will quickly turn into an unconscious routine.

Keep a close eye out for signs of dehydration, which can include:

Dry mouth or thirst
Dizziness
Faintness
Weakness
Light-headedness
Dry skin
Dark urine
Decreased urine output
Sleepiness
Sudden tiredness
Muscle weakness

If you experience any of these symptoms, contact your doctor right away.

Dumping

As soon as you start eating again after surgery, you will notice the difference in your "new" stomach, which now is a pouch. It's much smaller now, so it cannot handle as much food. It also cannot handle certain kinds of food, particularly right after surgery. Even drinks, whether flavored or plain old water, can cause problems. Everyone has his or her own ever-changing list of foods and drinks that work or don't work for them. For example, certain *brands* of water don't work for many. You may also find that you eat too fast or don't chew well enough or have swallowed air or take one bite too many.

Whichever factor it is, your system will remedy it by dumping. When one of the issues occurs and the pouch disagrees, your stomach will dump that food, still undigested, into the small intestine. Your body will react with one or a combination of the following:

Nausea
Vomiting
Diarrhea
Flatulence
Heart palpitations
Clamminess or sweating
Headaches

Some people may experience all of these symptoms. Others never experience dumping.

Dumping is not necessarily a bad thing. It's definitely not pleasant, but it's part of the tool of weight-loss surgery. After all, one dumping experience is all it usually takes to make you realize you don't want to do *that* again, whatever "that" was! You learn very quickly to pay attention to what you eat and drink as well as how fast or how much (see Chapter 5 for more information).

Dumping, if triggered, will typically come on immediately or in a relatively short time frame. There's another form, called late-stage dumping, that can happen hours after consuming the offending food or drink. Late-stage dumping typically involves these same symptoms but simply takes longer to happen. Of course, that makes it harder to keep track of exactly what caused it, which is another reason why keeping a food journal is critically important.

Diarrhea is fairly common after surgery. We hear many patients panic because they are experiencing loose bowels. Let's put it this way: liquids in, liquids out. If you aren't eating solids, this one is pretty self-explanatory, and some loosening of the bowels is to be expected. If it is excessive, however, let your doctor or nurse know.

Getting a Glimpse of Your Post-Op Stomach

What's it like to come home after the surgery? You feel good, but inside you know you are healing from major surgery. That new stomach—or, more accurately, pouch—of yours is going to need tender care for the first few months. You're healing from surgery and learning and developing new habits all at the same time. Your biggest jobs are trading in old ways of thinking for new ones and learning how to eat properly. (Chapter 5 outlines how you'll need to eat in the weeks following the surgery.)

Even if you usually heal quickly, never forget that you are having major surgery. The most important thing in the few days after is to rest and recuperate. Yes, you'll be up and walking around, but having peace and quiet to rest is most beneficial. Be sure to prepare your family and closest friends for this, too. If you only have the energy to spend time with your immediate family, let your friends and extended family know. They won't begrudge your taking it easy for a speedy recovery. You'll have plenty of time to be fast and furious when all that weight starts melting away and your energy level skyrockets!

———————— MAKING THE CONNECTION ————————

Laura's Story: This surgery has been an absolute lifesaver for me. Prior to surgery, at 320 pounds, it was an effort just to get up in the morning and get moving. By the time I got home from work, it was straight to the couch for me, as my back hurt so bad I could barely move. Between the backache and pain in both knees, it was terrible. I also had been on high blood pressure and cholesterol medication for years. The cholesterol medication was starting to elevate my liver enzymes, so I knew I had to make drastic changes in my life to get off these meds.

After lots of research into gastric bypass, and much encouragement from my mom (who went with me to the orientation for three different doctors), we both felt very comfortable with and settled on a surgeon. Getting through the process for surgery was easier than I thought, and before I knew it, I had a date set. I was so nervous, yet more excited at the same time, as I knew this surgery was going to give me back my life. The surgery itself was a breeze, as I had very little pain. The following three months were a little tougher, as I had to deal with lots of nausea, but I was OK with it because the weight was coming off, and fast!

I have lost a total of 135 pounds and have found new freedom I never knew I could have. I'm so addicted to cardio and working out that my life is centered around my physical activities. I am more outgoing than I have ever been in my life. It's such a joy to be able to do things with my son that I was never able to do when I was obese, such as riding every ride at theme parks, biking, and not feeling ashamed of who I am. I felt like I had been trapped in a turtle's shell, moving at a turtle's pace, and now I feel totally free. My new life has been an absolute blessing, and I wouldn't trade it for anything.

5

Learning How to Eat After Weight-Loss Surgery

If you ask a thousand different surgeons, you will get a thousand different eating-plan suggestions for those early weeks. There is no one right or wrong eating plan—the right one is the healthy one that works for you. It's the one that is easy on that new pouch, advances you slowly, and begins you on the road to making your own good choices. The information in this chapter is what has worked for us and for thousands in our groups, but I'm not advocating going against your doctor's suggestions. Your surgeon knows you and your situation and can tailor the plan specific to your needs. We find, though, that most surgeons and bariatric centers don't give out specific, individual plans but instead rely on a generalized plan as a guideline.

OVERCOMING THE FEAR OF FOOD

One woman, Nina, called me a month post-op. She was terrified. After meeting with her nutritionist, she thought she could never have a normal eating life again, not if she wanted to live. Yet she was really longing for spaghetti sauce. She'd been sticking with the broths and the soups. One day she was in a restaurant, and she took a bite of her sister's spaghetti sauce. Just the sauce, mind you. Well, that one bite sent her into such a panic that she went to the ladies' room and washed out her mouth. Then she called me because she thought she was going to die!

Another patient, Hamish, who'd lost 275 pounds, would get sick when his wife put his plate in front of him. It wasn't from eating something he knew his stomach couldn't tolerate, but because he was afraid of dumping (see Chapter 4). Nothing but fear was causing his dumping. His nutrition adviser made him think that the tiniest thing was going to trigger dumping and he would be in agony. Needless to say, food wasn't the real issue, and eventually he did learn that he could make healthy choices and eat appropriate portions without any issues.

This isn't to say that all nutrition advisers give bad advice. There are plenty of great ones out there. These professionals work with you to develop an eating strategy or guideline for you, specifically. Don't hesitate to ask your nutrition adviser questions—or even to question some choices they give you. If you feel a food isn't right for you, discuss it and work together to find alternatives. A nutrition adviser's objective is to develop a healthy eating plan that is going to carry you through this lifelong journey.

General Guidelines for the First Six Weeks After Surgery

People tend to make the post-op rules a lot more complicated than they really are. Yes, there are new rules to learn about what you can eat, how much, and how soon. Yes, you have to be careful. But don't panic! There is life after weight-loss surgery, and it's really not that complicated.

We've studied dozens of eating plans from different weight-loss surgery programs, and they all come down to three goals for your first six weeks.

- *Start with smooth, gentle foods.* Broths, then cream soups, then either soft foods or purees of "regular" foods will give your stitched and swollen stomach a chance to heal.
- *Eat twice as much protein as carbohydrates.* As my surgeon likes to tell his patients, "I'm going to say something now that you may not have heard before. I'm worried that you won't eat enough!" Enough protein, of course. The trick is to start with the protein first: the egg, the grilled fish, the cheese, and so on. Given your small pouch and diminished absorption rate, if you don't reach for proteins first, you run a greater risk of developing anemia and protein-related health issues.
- *Stay well hydrated.* Make sure to drink enough fluids. Here's one tip: set a timer on your stove, your cell phone, or your PDA to go off every 30 minutes. When it does, take a sip of water or another liquid like soup. Soon you will be in the habit of keeping well hydrated.

While you learn these rules, you'll begin to see how to take a more reasonable attitude toward what you eat. Keep in mind that we're just talking about food—follow some simple rules, and food won't do you any harm. It certainly won't kill you, unless you're allergic to it or it's tainted! We have lots of practical examples of regular people who find that the reasonable, livable attitudes toward food really do take hold.

In the past you've probably looked to food for emotional reasons—maybe for comfort or out of boredom, anger, loneliness, or stress. After surgery, your food focus will become more fuel related instead of emotion related. You can still enjoy good food, but you're enjoying good food *and* seeking out the best fuel for your body. It's not about eating just for the sake of eating. What a concept, huh? Food is your fuel, not your friend.

Keeping a food log or journal will really open your eyes to your eating habits. The "Keeping a Food Journal" section a bit later in this chapter will give you more information on how to do it.

Listening to Your Body's Signals

Have you ever eaten a cookie just because it was there? Have you seen a piece of pie or cake that just called out to you? You weren't hungry, but you ate it anyway. Or you ate one piece, and then another. Still, hunger wasn't involved, and your body sure didn't need all that sugar. It was pure emotional eating, whether for pleasure or anxiety, boredom or stress.

You now have to learn an entirely new way of looking at food. No longer can you just eat for the sake of eating. No longer can you eat until you're overstuffed. You're on the road to a whole new life. Throw out the old things you knew and used to do!

Most of us find that we've spent our entire lives ignoring any and all of our body's signals. Do you even remember what "full"

———————— MAKING THE CONNECTION ————————

Gilat's Story: My highest weight was 244 pounds, and at that point, I felt that there was nothing else I could do to lose the weight. I felt like I had tried every program out there, including all the pills available—both prescription and OTC—but the weight kept on finding me!

At the age of 31, I had a cholesterol level of over 300, and I kept gaining weight. I couldn't play outside with my kids. I didn't want to go out with my family since there was nothing that fit me well. I was size 20 or 22, and even that was getting tight on me. I hated the looks people gave me when I went grocery shopping, so I used the online services even for groceries. Everywhere I went, I felt like a second-class citizen, as though I wasn't good enough because I was too fat. I was sweating a lot, and even that was embarrassing! I even remember a time when I passed a car on the road and the driver was not pleased with that, so when he passed me back, he blew air into his cheeks and left them swollen to show me how fat I was. I would much rather have gotten the typical hand gesture than this reminder of how people see me.

I had no pictures of me with my kids. Not even one. My biggest fear was that I would die and my kids wouldn't have a picture of Mom to remember me by. Of course, even if I had one, did I really want them to remember me so fat and ugly?

I decided that this was just not the way to live! So I started my research. I read and read and read. I asked my physician for a surgeon referral. Then I called and attended a very informative seminar. Then came the psychological evaluation. I wasn't prepared at that time, and I was declined. But thank goodness, because this allowed me to spend the next few months getting to the right psychological point to succeed with this tool. Sure, it was frustrating to wait, and I even considered giving up. I wanted the surgery so badly that the rejection just added to my frustration. I am happy that I didn't give up, though. I persevered and followed my doctor's instructions. Then that wonderful letter finally arrived, the one that told me I am doing it, I am approved!

Then the nerves started to kick in. What if I failed? What if I died? But heck, if I died, at least I died trying! At least my kids would know that I had tried to do something to better my life and that I took a risk to make my life better.

Thank goodness I found a gastric bypass support group (http:// groups.msn.com/gastricbypasssupport), people who understood what I was going through and how to calm my nerves when they were a bit jittery. They knew to help me with new information, and, little by little, I learned how to share and help others, too. I was embarrassed at first to go through the surgery, but this group of people turned into a small online protective family who not only helped me through it but also cared about the outcome.

I was still scared the day of the surgery but by the time I woke up after, I already felt happy. Six weeks after the surgery, I was back to work, and before long, people were noticing me and the losses already. I am now 159 pounds and wearing size 8. Me? A size 8? I now go to the pool with my kids and enjoy life with them. I can't wait to go sledding with them this winter.

I also started going to school to take real estate classes! In the past, my weight prevented me from going after this goal because with a real estate license comes taking a picture, getting dressed in fancy clothes, and talking to many people. But now I'm not afraid of that. My husband, who said he never saw me as fat as I was, says that I look as good as when we met. He even calls me "exotic" sometimes. It feels great.

This surgery saved my life. This was not an easy journey, but it was well worth it. This is the most amazing tool our doctors can give us to start living life.

really feels like? Or do you equate being full with what is actually overfull? With this new stomach, you have to rely on weighing and measuring and concentration. You have to stop and think, "Am I really hungry?" before you eat. You have to learn what your fuel requirements are.

In the beginning of the post-op period, it's almost shocking the way you can forget to eat or drink. But it happens! The last thing you want to do, however, is to put your body in starvation mode, so it's very important to eat when your body needs the fuel. Setting a timer or finding your reminder point will help you to establish the habit.

When you do eat, you will now have to make choices you've never made before. You have to pay attention to what the food is,

NOTING THE CHANGE IN YOUR TASTE BUDS

After surgery, your tastes start to change. Things that were salty are *really* salty afterward. Things that were sweet are *really* sweet. You may even wonder how you ate some of these things before! At the same time, broths and really good water taste wonderful, with distinct flavors.

Many people notice that, before their surgeries, they had become almost impervious to flavors, mindlessly eating things over and over but not tasting them at all. We call this hypnotic eating. Have you ever driven somewhere and realized you don't remember part of the drive? It can be the same with eating. For example, sitting in front of a television, just snacking away without realizing you ate that whole bag of chips or cookies. Fast-forward beyond those days of mindless eating. Now instead of eating without thinking, you may find that you have to remind yourself to eat!

how much of it there is, what it contains, and more. I can't reiterate this enough. You even have to pay attention to the size of each bite and how many times you chew before swallowing.

Keeping a Food Journal

A food journal is a place not only for your thoughts and emotions (which will be cathartic for you in your weight-loss journey) but also for details about your food intake: what and how much you eat, when, and how your body reacted to those foods. You'll find a sample journal in Appendix B.

I can't tell you how happy you'll be that you kept a journal. Years after my surgery, I still go back through my journal and reread mine as a reminder of the stages and emotions I went through along the way. Every time I read it, I see something else that makes me pay closer attention to something I'm doing or otherwise make adjustments in my daily routine.

Many patients begin their journals with the process of obtaining surgery approval. As you research the surgery, your journal is an ideal place to keep a list of your questions and the answers you find. You'll also want to note your beginning weight and measurements, and perhaps store your "before" photos in your journal. Your journal is also a great spot for keeping up with appointments for lab work and doctors and more. It's a time capsule for you and will unfold your weight-loss journey before your very eyes.

In your food journal, you'll not only keep track of what you eat and drink but also trace the emotions that go with your eating patterns. It's an exercise in making you stop and really think about what you're eating and drinking and why. It doesn't take many days of keeping a food journal before you're actually *thinking* about your choices instead of eating absentmindedly, a habit that can bring big—as in added pounds—trouble.

Here are some tips for keeping your journal:

- Write down everything you eat and drink.
- Note how much you ate. Take the extra step to weigh and measure your foods, especially in the early days, so you'll truly understand portion sizes. Many patients learn that even one bite too much can trigger dumping. You need to see, not guess at, portion sizes.
- Keep details of how fast you eat and drink. Keeping this detail in your journal reminds you not to rush. Chew slowly and thoroughly. If you're swallowing a lump, you didn't chew well enough. Take small bites and pay attention to the way you're chewing and swallowing.
- Describe how your food tastes and what the texture was like. This is another exercise to help you pay attention to your food choices. These details also help you pinpoint foods that may be less satisfying or may trigger a grazing session as your body tries to find the taste it's really looking for.
- Note how the food made you feel. Did you eat to the "just right" amount for your pouch—not too full, but satisfied? Or did you dump from it? Did the food feel like it was a good fuel for your body? Did it make you feel more energetic? Or did it make you feel sleepy or otherwise bad? The effects of particular foods on you will change throughout your weight-loss journey. Recording this information will give you a guide to when such changes are occurring, which will help you adjust your intake to best suit to your body's needs.
- Record your emotions. Emotions play a big part in eating, and daily encounters and/or events can be pitfalls. Write them down, even if they seem completely unrelated to food. Whether it's an accomplishment or a difficult day, journaling the events will be therapeutic. Besides, journaling helps you

celebrate your achievements and learn from those pitfalls. It's a reference tool you'll utilize many times over.

■ Keep track of everything: questions; appointments; products, vitamins, supplements, and more that you want to check out or buy; your measurements; your weight; your goals; your feelings, accomplishments, and concerns; your food intake; before, in-process, and after photos; and so on.

The point is not only to make your journal reflect your personal journey but also to make it a tool to solidify your habits. You've gone so far in having major surgery, so take this extra step that will benefit you tremendously. Like so much of your life, you're developing new habits, and this is a great one. It's time to think new, fresh, and healthy!

Starting with Smooth, Gentle Foods

Because most weight-loss surgery patients recover quickly from the surgery itself, the post-op period is all about eating the right foods. Everyone's program is different, but six weeks seems to be a consistent time frame for the initial food progression. During this time, you have to remember your pouch is healing. For the first few weeks, it may be swollen and you may find that eating even 1 ounce of food makes you feel as if you've just had a full meal. Your new pouch has gone from the size of a football to about the size of an egg, so there are some major adjustments to make. Foods should be smooth and gentle—clear broths first; then creamier soups; then purees, soft proteins, and soft vegetables; and finally whole foods.

Beginning with Broths

Who would have thought that chicken broth, seafood broth, beef broth, or vegetable broth could be so delectable? Before surgery,

Dan and I could sit down and eat a big bowl of soup, but after surgery, it was a stretch for us to finish 2 ounces in 20 or 30 minutes. (Your eating habits won't stay that way forever, of course, but they do last for a considerable amount of time.) When we were allowed nothing but clear liquids the first week, we thought it was going to be miserable. But homemade broths never tasted so good. A little planning ahead really helped keep it easy for us, and I've shared some of my recipes in Appendix A. You can use these same recipes as a base for your cream soups as you move through your postoperative stages.

Making your own broth may be easier than you think. You don't have to use exact measurements, and there are so many variations, depending on your own tastes. So experiment and don't be surprised to find things you didn't like before surgery may now be some of your favorites. For example, we've known many people who didn't like fish before surgery who now find it to be their favorite food. If you've never had anything other than chicken broth, make vegetable, seafood, or beef broth. Use different seasonings or whatever vegetables are in season. Focus on both flavor and fresh ingredients. You control what goes into your broth, so you control the amount of sodium, the freshness, and the quality of your meal.

Most people find that during that first week, clear soups, 100 percent fruit juices, water, and protein drinks are the majority of their foods. Staying hydrated is so important, and clear soups and juices count in your daily fluid intake. Even at that, you may still find it takes some planning and thinking to get in that 64 ounces each day.

Adding Cream Soups and Purees

Dan and I are all about really good food and things with flavor. We tease each other that we are food snobs, because we just won't settle for mediocre. So when we reached the cream soup stage, we headed straight to one of our favorite restaurants for lobster bisque. All it took was dipping our spoons into it—just that one taste was as satisfying as eating an entire steaming bowl. One cup of soup was enough to last the two of us for several days— it was rich, flavor filled, and made with fresh ingredients. This equaled complete satisfaction for us. It also was the first time we realized just how important flavor and spices could be in our success, and it will be in yours, too.

After you have graduated from the cream soup stage, many patients go into the puree stage. Again, remember to think about flavor and moisture, and to take it slow and steady. For example, as you're pureeing fish or veggies, you can always roast foods first and then puree them. Instead of roasting one single vegetable, make up a combination of soft seasonal items so you have the freshest flavors. Consider adding a bit of cinnamon and Splenda to cottage cheese. Experiment with all sorts of foods, spices, and herbs! Remember, too, that your support group is a great source for ideas and suggestions on stage foods (see Chapter 4).

Moving on to Solid Foods

When it comes to solids, you want to keep easing in. Your new pouch is still adjusting to textures, and you don't want to rush. Try things like soft grilled fish or very moist chicken. I have to say, though, that chicken and eggs are some of the most common dumping offenders Dan and I hear about. There's no specific explanation for why these tend to be problem foods, but I have my own theory. Chicken and eggs can easily and quickly overcook. Because moisture content, density, texture, and tenderness are all factors in dumping, these foods have shown up on our "problem food complaint" list for fairly early post-ops. While they are not a problem for everyone, they do cause problems for many.

Make certain your solid foods are moist, or put them in some type of broth. Slow cookers (also called crock pots) are a weight-loss surgery patient's friend when it comes to keeping meats juicy and tender. If you haven't used one before, this is a great and inexpensive addition to your kitchen. A quick search on the Internet will turn up thousands of recipes, and any bookstore will have sections specifically for slow-cooker cooking. You'll also want to check out high-protein cookbooks and online recipes.

Eating Enough Protein

Your ultimate goal is to learn to reach for proteins first and good carbohydrates second. This is very difficult to achieve in the early weeks, prior to adding solid foods. But, with a little imagination and protein supplementation, it is quite possible. Ideally, across the board, the common recommendation for protein intake (at all stages) ranges from 60 to 90 grams per day. The body loses that much on its own, and it's particularly important that weight-loss surgery patients replenish that. After you move to whole foods, the usual recommendation is also a two-to-one protein-to-carb ratio. For example, if you eat 80 grams of protein in a day, then capping your daily carbohydrate intake at 40 grams will help continue the weight loss.

There's an unending supply of protein choices to be found. But, at least in the beginning, there are very few proteins that most weight-loss surgery patients like or tolerate well. In the early days of your postoperative period, you may want to use protein supplements, but the further you progress, the more protein you'll be able to get from your foods. Even later, however, some people still like to rely on protein supplements as meal replacements or just as an added boost to their day. Here are some of our favorite protein supplements:

- *ProFect protein drinks*: These are our favorite, because they are 2.9 fluid ounces with 25 grams of protein and *no* carbs or sugars. For more information, check out protica.com.
- *Unjury chicken soup*: This is a protein drink you mix and warm up, which is a nice switch from all of the sweet protein drinks. Find out more at unjury.com.
- *EAS AdvantEdge protein drink*: This protein drink can be purchased premixed at most mass merchandisers, health food stores, and pharmacies.
- *Isopure protein drink*: This protein drink can be purchased in premixed or mixable form.

As they progress, many people get into ruts, thinking protein means canned tuna, a piece of cheese, or eggs. Although those foods are fine and are good sources of protein, they can get old very quickly. A great suggestion for snacks is roll-ups, which is a way to stack your protein. For example, take a piece of thin-sliced turkey or ham, top it with cheese and bacon, and roll it up. That's stacking protein. Some of our favorite combinations include:

Ham, Jarlesberg cheese, deli mustard
Smoked turkey, fontina cheese
Smoked chicken, bacon, Gouda cheese
Smoked salmon, cream cheese, boiled egg, dollop of sour
  cream, a few capers
Roast beef, fontina cheese, horseradish-and-sour-cream
  sauce
Ham, scrambled egg, and cheese
Prosciutto, mozzarella, thin slice of cantaloupe
Turkey, pepper jack cheese, slice or two of avocado
Chicken, mozzarella, thin layer of marinara sauce for flavor
Ham, turkey, or chicken, with cream cheese and asparagus
  spear or pickle for crunch

Lettuce leaf, bacon, cheese, dab of mayonnaise
Lettuce leaf, shrimp, avocado or asparagus, cream cheese

The combination possibilities are endless. These combinations are also easy to have ready when that refueling urge hits and you don't have a meal prepared.

Staying Hydrated

Staying hydrated seems like a simple thing to accomplish. You'd be surprised how often we hear of patients who just don't feel like drinking, so they forgo their water or broth or clear juices. They begin feeling tired, but they write it off to having surgery and diminished food intake. Before you know it, they are in a hospital for IV rehydration!

Sipping, sipping, and more sipping throughout the day is something that needs to become a habit very quickly. Most programs suggest getting in 64 ounces of liquids per day. This 64 ounces includes the following:

Water
Clear, 100 percent fruit juices
Clear, nonsugared, noncarbonated, decaffeinated drinks
    (Crystal Light, Powerade, Propel, and so on)
Clear soups and broths

Note that sodas, even clear diet sodas, are completely out of the picture, for good (and for your own good!). In addition, caffeinated drinks such as coffee or tea can contribute to dehydration, so either avoid them or increase your fluid intake above what is normally recommended.

One very common thing we hear is how quickly patients get hooked on drinking water. What a great addiction! It's great for your skin and organs, helps keep your metabolism high, and flushes toxins out of the body. It's the perfect drink.

Checking for Vitamin Deficiencies

During the weeks and months following your surgery, you'll be starting on vitamins and supplements, seeing your surgeon for office vists, and having lab work done to identify possible vitamin deficiencies. It's important that you be proactive in your care. Yes, lab work is an additional step you didn't do on a regular basis before surgery. And maybe you didn't take vitamins regularly, either. But after the surgery, you are turning your focus to your health and are incorporating these new factors into your new life.

Most programs recommend taking a children's chewable vitamin or a sugar-free chewable vitamin for the first few weeks after surgery. They also recommend that you wait until approximately 30 days post-op to add in other supplements, such as vitamin B_{12}.

There's no need to buy specific brands or spend a small fortune on vitamins, so don't let someone convince you that you need to spend hundreds of dollars on products they are trying to sell you. Before taking any vitamins or supplements, however, talk with your pharmacist to make sure none of these will interact improperly with medications you are currently taking.

Vitamin Suggestions

Keep the following suggestions in mind when taking vitamins:

- Early post-op suggestions may include children's chewable vitamins, liquid vitamins, or some other approach. Flavor can be a factor, so keep your receipt in case you need to make a return and find a different product that works for you and tastes decent enough to take every day.

■ Once you're past the early weeks, most patients find that a good multivitamin or prenatal vitamin (chelated for better absorption) are quite acceptable.

■ When taking calcium, look for calcium citrate, not calcium carbonate. Be sure to read labels, as many calcium supplements are large *and* require you to take five or six pills to meet your daily requirements. Take calcium citrate alone (at least two hours after any other vitamins or supplements) and in doses of no more than 600 milligrams each. The typical daily suggested amount is 1,200 to 1,500 milligrams per day. Rely on your lab results (in consultation with your surgeon) for adjustments to meet your individual needs.

■ Vitamin B_{12} is a requirement for life for weight-loss surgery patients. Acceptable forms are sublingual, nasal spray, or intramuscular injection. Don't use insulin needles for these injections due to potential tissue damage if the injection isn't deep enough.

Lab Work

Lab work, which tests your B_{12} and other levels, such as TIBC (total iron binding capacity), vitamin D, calcium, and more, is a must for weight-loss surgery patients. Usually, the panels (types of tests) done on your blood will include CBC (complete blood count), liver panel, lipid panel, iron, chem-12 (a panel with 12 different lab values), beta-carotene, and more. Your doctor will determine which types of test you'll need and how often, but most patients have lab work done at one month, three months, and six months post-op, and then annually for life. This testing isn't something to ignore or neglect. Simple tests can allow for quick adjustments before you experience any negative side effects of vitamin deficiencies. It can also provide reassurance that the vitamins and supplements you are taking are the right ones.

───────────── MAKING THE CONNECTION ─────────────

Lauren's Story: I have been overweight my entire life. As far back as I can recall, my mother would put her arm around my shoulder and introduce me to her friends like this: "This is my daughter, Lauren, and to think, she was my *smallest* baby." Throughout my teens, she made sure I was on what seemed like every diet that ever came out.

When I was about 12, I was actually "thin": I was 5'8" and weighed 135 pounds. Circumstances arose, though, and I began to gain. Then more dieting and the yo-yo of gaining and losing. This continued until I ballooned up to over to 300 pounds at one point.

At the age of 48, my health was poor. My blood pressure, cholesterol, and triglycerides were out of control. My blood sugars were over 300 on a good day. My diabetes was killing me. The medications I took couldn't work because I couldn't control myself enough to eat properly. I lost the feeling in some of my toes. I was scared . . . but not scared enough.

At one point a coworker friend came to me and said she was considering gastric bypass surgery. She never pressured me but came often to my office and shared what she was learning about the surgery and the process. One day, she said that after surgery you aren't allowed caffeine or carbonation. I told her then that surgery was out for me. There wasn't any way I could give up my 12-pack-a-day habit of diet cola. But I thought about it daily on my drive to and from work and decided that if I could give up the soda, that maybe I could be disciplined enough to have surgery. And I was!

I decided to have surgery because I *wanted* to live long enough to watch my girls graduate and walk down the aisle at their weddings, and I wanted to be able to hold my grandchildren and tell them tales about their mothers. I want to grow old with the man I love and sit beside him, rocking together on the front porch.

I had my surgery and have lost a total of 110 pounds. I am a success. That is not an easy thing for me to say out loud, because I still see the "fat" girl in the mirror, but I am working on that mental image. I am healthy. I do not take any prescription medicines and haven't since the day of my surgery. I have a new lease on life. I can tie my shoes without thinking my face is going to pop off my head because I am squishing all my fat together. Although I still despise shopping, it is a lot easier to find clothes that I can fit into. I lost a shoe size. Considering that I used to wear a men's size 11, this is a good thing.

I believe I have more confidence in myself. I used to fake that a lot before but now I no longer need to. I can walk and exercise without my thighs rubbing together and catching on fire. So, Smokey, I am doing my part to prevent forest fires! And, obviously, I haven't lost my "fat girl" sense of humor.

My relationship with my husband is rich and full. We are able to do more things together since my surgery. We kayak, go to the gym, and do other things I would have never done before because of my weight. Even though my husband never complained about my weight, he loves the thinner, happier, healthier me.

I could not have gone through with the surgery without the love and support of my family and friends.

Do I have any regrets at all? I have only one. It would be that I didn't have the surgery many years ago. There are a lot more things that I am grateful for, but what I am saying is that I thank God every day for giving me the chance to have gastric bypass surgery and be healthy again.

Eating Outside the Home: Handling Restaurants and Parties

At home, you can be in control of what foods you have around you. But what happens to your new relationship with food when you start eating at restaurants, attending parties, and going to or hosting holiday dinners?

Wait . . . did you read that right? Restaurants? Parties? Can you really have delicious food? You bet you can!

Weight-loss surgery doesn't preclude you from eating out. Instead, it puts you in a position to be more selective in what you do consume. Some people are afraid to eat for fear of returning to their old self or their old ways. But eating has many components, and, although your relationship with food does change dramatically, your attachment to food and the joys of eating won't go away after weight-loss surgery.

Dan and I say we're food snobs because we love—and I do mean love—a great meal, and we choose not to settle for eating mediocre meals. At first, we thought we were going to have to mourn our old friend, food, and put an end to our dining-out experiences. We couldn't have been more wrong.

RESTAURANT CARD

Many surgical programs offer a restaurant card that gives a basic overview of what the patient has had done and his or her need for reduced portions. Although most restaurants don't require the card or even ask for them, it's a handy thing to carry with you. Following is an example of the card text:

Special Diet Request
Holder of this card, Firstname Lastname, is a gastric
    bypass patient of:
Dr. Firstname Lastname
1234 Street Name, City, State 12345
XXX-XXX-XXXX

This patient has undergone gastric bypass surgery by the listed surgeon, which has reduced his/her stomach capacity to less than 3 ounces. Please allow him/her to order a smaller portion or make a selection from the children's menu.

We offer this card free of charge; send a stamped, self-addressed envelope with a note including your e-mail address to The Weight-Loss Surgery Connection, 1971 W. Lumsden, Ste. 250, Brandon, FL 33511.

Just because you're eating less doesn't mean that you're not eating at all or that you can't celebrate eating and still be in control. Good food and good company go hand in hand in social settings, and you and your small pouch don't have to miss out. In fact, Dan and I appreciate good food and good company even more now that we've had our surgeries. Our awareness of the foods we're eating is heightened, which tends to make social settings even more enjoyable. Flavors and smells take on a whole new dimension, something you'll likely notice soon after your surgery. Even the most delicate nuances in taste, texture, and visual presentation are apparent.

Whether dining out or cooking in, the trick to eating successfully with others is to learn to enjoy the social factor first and to make the food secondary. No more will you tuck your head down and eat for an hour, gobbling up one course after another. No more will you check out the dessert menu first because you're saving room for something sugary sweet. Those days of mindless noshing are no more. Instead, you'll find a whole new way to enjoy the social aspects of your meal. And when you're done eating, you won't feel bloated and miserable like you used to, either. You'll feel great and in control of your eating and your choices.

Ultimately, food is just food. It's not entertainment. It's not ever going to love you back, make you laugh, or give you comfort when you're sad. By focusing on the social aspects of eating, as well as the nutritional components, you can enjoy your friends or the setting more. You're feeding the spirit instead of just filling the pouch.

At the same time, food will still be something you can and will enjoy. Who doesn't enjoy an exceptional meal? Flavors, aromas, and beautiful presentation are rolled into delicious morsels before us. The key is remembering that you control what you eat. You control your choices and your portions. You're looking for those morsels instead of mountains of food to taste and savor and sustain you.

Eating in Restaurants

If you're like many morbidly obese individuals, eating out can seem intimidating, even overwhelming at times. But after weight-loss surgery, the picture changes considerably. No more are you going to sit down and order three or four courses and eat mindlessly. The meal will now be partially about refueling, but even more about visiting with friends, family members, or coworkers. When you relax and start talking and sharing with others, the focus comes off of the food. If this idea seems hard to picture, don't worry—having a comfortable dining experience is not so much a challenge as it is a relearning experience.

We go out to dinner once a month with our support groups, and we show them how to prepare for a good experience, including how to order. Eating out doesn't have to be an ordeal, but you do have to be more selective in your choices and requests.

There are three challenges to eating out after weight-loss surgery:

- How to get the right kind of food from the waitstaff
- How to get the right amount of food from the waitstaff
- How to find new ways to enjoy the social aspect of the meal

In this section, I help you address these issues and develop healthy habits for the challenges and pleasures of eating away from home.

Getting Enough Protein

First, you will need to find new ways to get enough protein. Look for grilled fish, meats, poultry, and so on. Many restaurants have added low-carb sections to their menus and offer high-protein fare that is quite tasty and healthy. If you don't see anything on the menu that's grilled, pan seared, or sautéed, ask whether your server can bring you some kind of protein that isn't fried or coated in sauces.

You may discover that some of your old favorites aren't your favorites anymore. Pasta, for example, will have to become a very rare side dish, because even a small entree of pasta turns your new stomach into a lead balloon. Many restaurants have sides of grilled or steamed vegetables available, or you might order a small salad.

Getting the Proper Portion Size

Typical restaurant portions these days are about three times what you need for your meal. Even the "smaller" portions served by some restaurants are still way more food than you can or want to consume. This means you'll likely have to ask for a specific portion size. We frequent some restaurants that will weigh out a 2-ounce portion of fish or cut a 2- or 3-ounce piece of steak. It's not unreasonable to ask for and expect such service.

Dan and I travel quite a lot and eat many meals in restaurants. Out of the thousands of restaurants we have frequented, very few have ever refused to be accommodating in our specific requests. From the time the server begins taking our order, we fill him or her in on our individual requirements—that's just how we like to approach our experiences dining out. Servers are usually extremely helpful, wanting to do anything they can to make certain our needs are met. Don't be afraid to speak up for yourself regarding portion size, even if in the past you tended to be a wallflower and felt uncomfortable speaking up for yourself. Just practice a bit and give yourself some time, and you will get better—and far more comfortable—with stating your needs.

You have to decide how much you want to divulge, but most people are fascinated with our having had this procedure—and our success. Eating out is just one more venue for us to share our story and, perhaps, help someone else along the way. We are so proud of our life changes, we never miss an opportunity to talk about how weight-loss surgery has changed and saved our lives.

We're very open about what we've had done. We carry before and after photos everywhere we go and share them openly. Usually, the server has to call over another server, the manager, and anyone else within earshot. All become wowed by the changes. Even people sitting at nearby tables tend to be drawn into the conversation. As a result, total strangers quickly become attached and begin making sure things are just right for us. We've gone from being unwanted, morbidly obese, invisible individuals to people others can connect with. What begins as a simple meal ends with our making new acquaintances and learning something about them as well.

We look at this sharing in more than one way. One, it helps us out by meeting our own small-portion needs, but at the same time we share the positives of weight-loss surgery. Just because the people we are speaking to are not morbidly obese, odds are they know or love someone who is. So there we sit, prime examples of what works about this surgery and why. We're educating others along the way and, with any luck, making it a little easier for the next weight-loss surgery patient who visits that restaurant.

This may not sound like your ideal dining experience, but it's quite pleasant for us, and thousands of weight-loss surgery patients have shared similar stories with us. If it matches your personality, don't be afraid to speak up for yourself or to share. People really are more kind and caring than you might think.

When ordering, we typically start off with an abbreviated version of our story, or just the fact that we've both had gastric bypass and can eat only very small portions. Dan tends to explain that our stomachs have gone from the size of a football to the size of an egg. Some establishments will ask for our restaurant card, but most don't even require them and accommodate easily.

With limited real estate in your stomach, you want to make certain that what you put in that tiny pouch is both delicious and nutritious—flavor and quality over quantity. A child's menu is not the answer, because the food choices on those menus typically aren't the healthiest and certainly aren't high protein. You could probably split a serving with a friend, but chances are that your friend will not want to split a portion, nor will you both want to eat the same thing. You need to order smaller portions from the regular menu,

One of two things usually happens when you ask for a small portion: either the server understands and begins offering suggestions, or he or she instinctively says no to the smaller portions. A negative answer isn't acceptable! Any good restaurant that cares about its customers is not going to begrudge your having a smaller portion. If a server does the instinctive no, calmly ask to speak with a manager. Generally, when the manager arrives at the table, we give a brief explanation, and he or she becomes quite helpful. Most managers will accommodate you. If not, it's your option to stay or to leave the restaurant and go elsewhere. There are plenty of great restaurants out there that want your business. You won't be making a scene; you're just expecting true customer service.

Why do you need to ask for a smaller portion? Well, you now have this tiny little pouch, so there's no need for such big portions and no need to pay full price for meals you know you can't even come close to finishing. Why be so wasteful with so much food? Even a half portion is more than the typical weight-loss surgery patient can consume. Not only are you going to receive a smaller portion, which is still more than you can consume, but your dining bill should be reduced as well. Each restaurant has its own way of applying discounts, whether it's half price, kid's price, half price with a slight add-on, or whatever scale they set. We've never had a single restaurant refuse to reduce pricing when the portion was reduced. Now you're not only eating less, but you're spending less, too!

Did you know that many restaurants already have reduced lunch portions but will even cut those in half? We frequent some of the chain restaurants that have proved to be quite accommodating. Such restaurants as Bahama Breeze, Olive Garden, Smokey Bones, Bonefish Grill, Carraba's, Macaroni Grill, Sam Seltzer's, Red Lobster, and many more gladly prepare half portions of anything on their menus. We spoke with their corporate offices before we started dining out and were told that these restaurants would absolutely work with every customer's needs. We've definitely found this to be true.

What a lot of restaurants realize is that most weight-loss surgery patrons are going to bring other patrons along as well. Odds are you'll have others with you (friends, family, coworkers) who are eating full portions, so they are not losing money. But even if

MAKING FRIENDS WITH RESTAURANT PERSONNEL

If you need to ask a manager for assistance and you otherwise enjoy your visit to that restaurant, get the manager's name and use it throughout the conversation. You'll make a friend there, which means that asking for small portions at that restaurant shouldn't be an issue again. You may even want to follow up with a note after the meal. Also, if a server has been particularly kind or obliging, go to the restaurant's website and send a nice compliment or fill out a comment card, if available. These may seem like little things, but we've made friends at restaurants all across the country this way.

you don't have others with you, still expect to receive the portion you need. Don't be bashful. Put your fear aside. Put your health and your needs first. It really is OK for you to speak up and ask for what you need. Once you realize there's nothing to fear, dining out can become a pleasant experience for you.

If you don't feel comfortable asking for a smaller portion while eating out, ask the server to divide your meal in half, with one half served now and the other put into a take-out container. Or you can ask to have a take-out container delivered when your meal is delivered. Before you take the first bite, put that extra portion away. Finally, you can just ask for an extra plate. You can still divide out your own small serving and ask for a take-out container at the end of the meal.

Use the journal pages in Appendix B to jot down your favorite restaurants, the names of staff or managers who were particularly helpful, specialties you enjoyed and want to try again, and anything else you want to remember from your dining-out experience.

Getting Creative When Ordering

Instead of looking at the menu as a whole, you will soon find that there are ample components you can put together if you want to order quickly and not discuss your surgery. While we love discussing the surgery, you may want to go in, order, and enjoy your meals. If that sounds like you, here are a few suggestions:

- Look at appetizers that can be a tasty entree. Items such as fresh ahi tuna, grilled shrimp, and grilled chicken skewers make great small entrees (although they are usually still too much food). When in doubt, ask your server about the portion sizes.
- Look for items that aren't breaded or coated in sauces, or ask the server for recommendations. If there are sauces, ask for

them to be placed on the side so you can test your tolerance as well as control how much you are ingesting.

■ Check out the side dishes or side salads as a complement to your entree. Most restaurants offer a side salad or cup of soup for a reduced price.

■ Ask about seasonal vegetables. Crisp, fresh vegetables are not only healthy but are typically readily available in most restaurants. Also check the children's or senior's menu for delicious vegetable plates in very small portions. More and more restaurants are making these smaller offerings available.

■ Consider the soup of the day. Our favorite Thai restaurant, Jasmine Thai, for example, offers a different soup each day as a side to their regular lunch menu and in a much reduced portion. This, along with a small side of steamed dumplings (one dumpling for each of us), makes for an excellent and flavorful meal. Before surgery, we would have started off with the soup and the dumplings and then made our way through a full entree and sides. Now, we're quite satisfied with the small portions and the variety we find on a regular basis. Variety keeps us from getting into food ruts as well.

Tapping Tapas Restaurants

For variety, a great restaurant option is a tapas restaurant, which offers small (appetizer size) portions that you can share with your friends. Tapas restaurants are perfect for weight-loss surgery patients, but they are extremely popular with nonsurgery folks, too.

Tapas restaurants are Spanish in origin, but the flavors are from around the globe. The idea behind these delectable restaurants is a selection of small, flavorful morsels to be shared with others. A variety of meats, cheeses, spices, and oils are preva-

--- MAKING THE CONNECTION ---

Doris's Story: When I was morbidly obese, I felt I had no control. I didn't have "only" 10 or 20 pounds to lose—I had almost 200 pounds to lose! It was a very sad way to live, because I felt there was no way out. I would cry all the time and felt I was trapped. I didn't want to go to social events with my husband because I felt bad for him, so either I'd send him alone, or neither of us would go and we would just make up an excuse why we couldn't make it. You can't really say, "Sorry I can't make it, because I'm so ashamed of myself that I wouldn't be comfortable, but thanks for asking."

I felt bad for my kids, too. I wasn't able to be active with them, and I was afraid of causing embarrassment for them when they needed me at school. Something that hurts your kids just kills you.

My first impression of surgery was I would never go through anything like that, because it was too dangerous and too scary. But I was very uninformed about it. As I gained and I reached 300 pounds, and then 310, 320, 330, I knew I had to find any and all options, given that I had high blood pressure, sleep apnea, and depression. I knew I couldn't do it on my own, though.

I researched all the different options, read books, searched the Internet, and felt that Roux-en-Y was the "tool" I needed to be successful. I had fears, but I knew that this was going to save my life and give me many more years—healthy years—to enjoy my life. I knew that, sooner or later, I would die due to complications from being morbidly obese, and I was not giving up without a fight.

I was excited, scared, anxious, worried, happy, nervous, so I joined my other "family" on gastricbypasssupport@groups.msn .com. My online family has been there, done that, so I asked questions, lots and lots of questions. Hearing answers from people who have gone through what I was about to go through really helped!

I had my surgery, and so far, in my first seven months, I'm down 120 pounds, from 332 to 212. I am in control of food; food no longer controls me!

My life has changed in so many wonderful ways. I feel great! I feel proud, and not only for me but because I'm not embarrassed for my family any longer. I don't feel sad or trapped anymore . . . I feel free, energized, and full of life!

---

lent in tapas dishes. Items such as fish and fresh seafood are traditional tapas staples and fill your high-protein needs. When paired with spices, healthy oils, and small portion sizes, the flavorful foods at tapas restaurants satisfy even the most picky palate.

Making Friends with Sushi Bars

A sushi bar is probably my all-time favorite food form. If the thought of eating raw fish doesn't appeal to you, many American versions of sushi are cooked. In addition, sushi uses a very high-quality grade of fish, which is packed with protein. So you're getting the freshest fish, in small portions. You may even find a sushi chef who is willing to make custom orders for you or to offer suggestions for the freshest catch of the day. And there's nothing wrong with asking your sushi chef to make you a roll with no rice (called a sashimi roll) or to cut your pieces extra small or cut them in half. This is another great way to get variety in small bites.

There are many great dining-out choices. Don't give up your healthy favorites just because you eat a smaller amount now.

Hosting a Party

Dan and I are passionate about cooking, and we want everyone who comes to our home to enjoy themselves. Contrary to what people may think when they get an invitation to our house, we don't do low-fat anything, because carbohydrates have replaced the fat in most low-fat items. The last thing we want is hidden carbs, when good fats and proteins in foods make you feel full longer.

When we prepare a party or celebration feast or even just a neighborhood get-together, no one feels deprived. We don't presume to expect everyone to eat like we do, so we make certain there's a wide variety of foods to fit everyone's tastes. That includes us—we have a bite here or there over the course of the day.

And thanks to our new sense of taste and smell, the food smells are so intense that it's almost as if we've eaten an entire meal without taking a single bite. You may laugh and think, "I wish I could feel full without actually eating!" But it's very true, and it's a big part of the post-op life. The sense of smell is so heightened after surgery that even to this day, if we go into a restaurant or a home where there are strong food smells, it can trigger a dumping episode. Who would have thought you could get overfull just by smelling something?

It's funny how people can react when you are planning a party or get-together. Chances are, at some point, you'll encounter a not-so-gracious friend or relative who makes a rude comment about what you will serve. Just this year, a member of our support group was approached by a relative who was concerned over what the weight-loss surgery patient was going to serve at a holiday meal, expecting that only things like beef jerky and cheese and protein drinks would be served. Not only was this a ridiculous assumption, but it was hurtful to our friend, who had diligently prepared a delectable menu of goodies for all her guests and was conscientious about their individual needs as well as her own. If you find yourself in that situation, just suggest that the individual bring whatever he or she feels comfortable eating. Put it back on him or her and don't let a spoiler kill your fun. In the end, a gathering of family and friends should be enough on its own, without food being the focus of the event.

When planning a dinner party or potluck gathering, remember to consider those who haven't had weight-loss surgery in addition to meeting your own nutritional needs. When Dan and I throw a party, we opt to do it one of two ways. We may include a menu along with our invitation, to avoid any undue questions or concerns from our guests. Or we may prepare the main dish proteins and ask guests to bring a side dish or dessert of their choosing. Either way, you can alleviate any stress or fear on the part of your guests.

We also stress that the point of the gathering is socializing with friends and/or family. Taking the focus off the food and placing it on our friends and family members shows them that they are important to us and that the food is secondary to their company and conversation. Isn't that what parties should be about anyway?

Attending Someone Else's Party

How do you handle going to someone's home and not knowing whether there will be anything there you can eat? Plan ahead for yourself. You might ask the host or hostess what type things they'll be serving and if you can bring a dish. More than likely, the host or hostess will give you a hint at what type foods will be served.

Most party hosts serve some type of protein (cheese, shrimp, meat), and you can eat small portions of these. If protein won't be served, eat before you go and pack yourself a cooler of your favorite bottled water. You might even bring a light snack (one that you can break away to eat, if needed) or a protein shake. Would you be upset if someone was watching out for their specific needs while a guest in your home? Of course not, and most

———————— MAKING THE CONNECTION ————————

Kathy Jo's Story: I've had weight issues all my life. I was the fat girl in first grade who was never picked to be on anyone's teams and was laughed at because my clothes were not stylish (they didn't make stylish clothes for chubby kids back then). Needless to say, these traumatic experiences led to a lifetime of low self-esteem and additional weight problems. In college, I developed eating disorders that included starvation, taking laxatives, binge eating, and so on.

After marrying and having two children, my weight went out of control. In my thirties, I did once get control and lose 50 pounds and was at my goal weight. I worked for Weight Watchers and kept my weight off for five years. But then again the old childhood voices played in my mind: I'm not good enough, I could weigh less, my body still doesn't look good! With these tapes playing in my mind, one day I was 5 pounds over my goal, and then it seems I turned around and I was 25 pounds over goal! A few years later, totally out of control, I was 75 pounds heavier. All the while, the tapes played in my mind, saying, "I told you that you couldn't do it."

Then the health issues began: the muscle aches, the joint aches, the flulike symptoms. Shortly after, I had a diagnosis of lupus that was treated with high doses of prednisone. Add on another 25 pounds and my life was essentially over: no playing with the kids, no going out with friends, no sexual relationship with my husband, and still the tapes playing in my mind I wasn't good enough. My life was out of control physically as well as mentally.

I found myself having a nervous breakdown and being admitted to a psychiatric unit for a week. I was now 110 pounds overweight and at my lowest mentally. I began to think about and look into this surgery, but it took me another year to decide it was time to get control of my mind, soul, and body.

It has been a year since my surgery, and I weigh 118 pounds less (the lowest in my adult life). I have a normal BMI, my muscles are now under control, I am off prednisone, I can walk a flight of stairs, and I can be a normal person with a normal clothes size. But most important, the talk in my mind has stopped.

For me, the surgery taught me to eat good healthy food, follow the program as it is written, and not try things that are not good for me! I can't tell you what a blessing it has been for my life!

---

people will feel the same way when you're visiting their homes. I'm not suggesting that you become a closet eater or sneak off to grab snacks stowed in your car. What I am suggesting, though, is to be prepared and proactive about your own needs. Your life is different from someone who hasn't had weight-loss surgery. Your energy level can drop quickly when that tiny little pouch reaches the empty mark on your body fuel gauge.

Slow Food

Have you ever stopped to really taste your food? In the past, when dining out, you may have been talking and eating until, before you know it, the food was gone and dessert was on the way. What did that entree taste like? What about the veggies? What types of seasonings were used? Were the sauces or flavors ones that you particularly enjoyed?

Take a look around sometime and observe the amount of food people put into their mouths. Dan and I marvel at people who eat, in one bite, almost as much as our entire pouches will hold. But how can you really taste—and enjoy—your food unless you take your time and focus on each bite?

A better strategy is to taste every bite like it's the first bite, as though you've been waiting for something delicious and know your mouth is going to be filled with the flavors you love. Take it

PRIORITIZING

Do you see a consistent thread throughout this book? It's about *you*. It's OK to make you and your needs a priority. It doesn't mean you're being self-centered or putting anyone else on the back burner. It does mean you are seeing the value of yourself and how that value is warranted. After so many years of devaluing yourself, this is quite a change of events and is a relearning process, just like relearning how to eat or what to do after surgery.

slowly. Make every bite one to be savored. Take a bite, and then put your fork down. If the food is something you particularly like, can you detect what is in the combination of flavors? Chew that bite until it's well chewed, and then swallow. Don't have your fork poised with the next bite before you've consumed the current one. Slow, slow, slow. Taste, taste, taste. If it's a good-quality meal, it's worth savoring anyway. You have only so much space for each meal, so why rush through it?

Do you find it odd that I'm talking so much about eating and about various foods? There is a method to my madness! Food doesn't disappear from your life after weight-loss surgery. Your focus changes dramatically, of course, but you learn to appreciate food and utilize it in a whole new light. Food is no longer the center of your world, but it is still something you will enjoy immensely.

Dining isn't just a pleasant experience; it will now be a *new* experience for you. Every aspect of your eating habit will change, but we think you're going to be pleasantly surprised when you dine out or host guests in your home. Look at each dining experience as something you can learn from. Learn something new about the person you're with or share something new about you. Learn a new flavor combination or ask about spices you don't recognize. Learn a favorite server's name or a manager's name. Dining should turn out to be far easier than you expected.

Speak up. Speak out. Ask for what you want, and expect to receive it. I think you'll be pleasantly surprised by the responsiveness and your own renewed ability to watch out for someone very important: you.

───────────── MAKING THE CONNECTION ─────────────

Robin's Story: I started to gain weight at the age of 12. My mother somehow felt that ridicule would get me to lose weight. If I ran down the stairs, she would yell, "*Walk* down those stairs, thunder thighs." She would call me El Chubs, and she would tell me that if I gained any more weight she would have to take me to Tilly the Tentmaker to buy my clothes. The ridicule I received at school was bad enough, but to hear it from my mom was the worst.

At 23, I had my son, and I weighed 240 pounds after his birth. I had tried every diet on the planet, and although I had yo-yo'd, the lowest I weighed was 193. I developed type 2 diabetes, but that didn't stop my poor eating habits. I just figured the meds would take care of it. They didn't. On top of that, I smoked. Eventually, I had a coronary episode and a stent placed, and still I didn't change.

Finally, I decided it was time to seek out counseling. I took a good hard look at my self-destructive behavior and eventually realized that I was going to be dead if I didn't do something. I quit smoking, but then I ballooned to 270 pounds. Diets just weren't working, and I needed to do something more drastic, so I looked into weight-loss surgery. I decided that was what I needed. I was already changing my eating habits and I knew that, with surgery, I would have a tool I could use.

I had the surgery just a short time ago, and I already feel like a new woman. In the first two weeks alone, I lost 22 pounds. I am very excited and positive and have found that my online support group has given me so much help and incentive. I know that I can do this. The thin girl inside that has been screaming to be set free is on her way out. I won't need Tilly the Tentmaker to make clothes! I have a sense of humor about that now.

I continue to research the weight-loss surgery process and gather healthy recipes. I also look at food differently now. I don't need it to comfort me. I don't need it to be my drug of choice. I need it to sustain a healthy life. My life is starting over, and I am so grateful that I have the opportunity to lead the life I always wanted.

Continuing to Lose Weight: Overcoming Obstacles to Progress

As Dan and I walked through a large department store one day, I suddenly realized that I was about to walk right out of my underwear. I'm not talking about my underwear being a little loose. Instead, I had recently lost so much weight that I was experiencing full-fledged, dropping to the knees, oh-my-gosh-who-is-looking, my underwear is falling off my body! If I'd been wearing a skirt, I would have just walked right out of them and kept going.

I had lost a dramatic amount of weight, but I hadn't even realized it. Poor Dan didn't have a clue what was going on as I rushed him out of the store. All I kept saying was, "We have to leave. We have to leave. We have to leave," and he said I was walking with my knees clinched and taking tiny little steps. I laugh about it now, but I was stunned when it happened. You expect pants and shirt sizes to change, but you forget about things like your underwear or your shoe size.

This story illustrates that your mind may have trouble keeping up with your body. The gap between thoughts and reality make for a funny story, but it also illustrates a serious threat to your progress. When it comes to losing weight, you have to exercise your *mind* as well as your body. The morbidly obese usually have years of disappointment, frustration, and unhelpful thought patterns behind them, and our minds aren't usually ready, at first, to appreciate or sustain the amazing success we can achieve after surgery.

There are many mental traps and other obstacles that can put your progress in danger, and recognizing them—as well as knowing how to take action when you hit them—is an important step toward making sure the weight keeps falling off. In this chapter, I discuss the major obstacles you'll face, as well as some solutions to keep your progress on track.

Gauging Your Expectations

New weight-loss surgery patients often make the mistake of trying to base their own weight-loss expectations on the results of others. Many new patients want to know how much they will lose, how fast they'll lose, what the average is, when they will be at their goal weight, how soon they'll be at work—more, more,

more, faster, faster, faster. This intensity can build motivation and enthusiasm, but it can also border on dangerous when people get too tied to a number.

It's normal to want to know what to expect, but keep in mind that there are many variables. For one thing, men tend to lose weight faster than women because they have more muscle mass. Here's an example: Dan and I both had surgery on the same day, with the same surgeon. We followed the exact same plan and the same eating and drinking schedule. Would it be realistic for me to expect to lose the same amount of weight at the same pace as Dan? No. Dan had a higher starting weight than I did: his 400 pounds to my 264 pounds was a substantial difference. He's 13 inches taller and six years older than I am, both of which also came into play. In a mere eight months, we both achieved our goal weights, but those goal weights were very different. His loss was 180 pounds to my 120 pounds. If I had lost 180 pounds like he did, I would weigh 84 pounds!

There are other factors. Each surgeon varies the size of the pouch and how much small intestine is bypassed. Both can be key factors in the speed with which one loses weight. Couple that with what you eat, when, how often, and how much, not to mention your water intake or your activity levels, and you can see how many variables there are.

Just because you have surgery doesn't mean you'll experience magical numbers. The success of weight-loss surgery comes from relearning how to eat, not from the surgery itself. I know of one woman who insisted she could have the surgery, make no changes in her life, and lose 150 pounds in five months. Wouldn't we all love something like that? But that's just not a reality. The potential is there to lose the weight, but your primary objectives are to *keep* the weight off, get yourself permanently out of a high-risk category, and become as healthy as you can possibly be!

When you meet with your surgeon, sit down and discuss expectations. No one knows your situation better than your surgeon—your medical history as well as the procedure being performed and what to anticipate in your specific case.

You are going to lose weight. Maybe you'll lose twice what I did, or half of what I did, in the same time frame. The good news is that you're losing weight, you're making the changes you need to make, and you're going to keep losing. See that as winning, however much you lose.

Anticipating Plateaus

One day, the number on the scale will stop going down. You're eating right, you're getting exercise, but you're not losing any more weight. If you allow yourself to panic, you'll be plagued with self-doubt and questions like, "What am I doing wrong?" You may even be tempted to take drastic measures.

Don't.

Plateaus—those times during which weight loss will level off for a while—*will* happen. They're inevitable, and they will happen more than once. Every single weight-loss surgery patient can tell you they've hit plateaus. You have to prepare yourself and understand that plateaus are just part of the process.

It's common to experience your first plateau around your fourth week after the surgery. Our doctor told us the body needs a break to catch up with its rapid weight loss. A plateau can last for a few days, a week, several weeks, or even a month or more. Regardless of how long it lasts, it can become very discouraging if you let it. You may feel that your new habits aren't working and be tempted to give them up.

Instead, consider staying away from the scale for a few days during a plateau. Remember that, throughout your postsurgery weight loss, you're recording not only your weight but also your measurements. Measurements are just as important as weight, so when you're still losing inches and making progress—regardless of what's happening on the scale—let that keep you motivated until the numbers start heading down again on the scale.

Think of plateaus as a time to review what you're doing. Perhaps it is a plateau, or perhaps your food choices are causing the slowdown. Maybe you're doing things exactly right, or maybe it's time to make some small adjustments in what you're eating

WEIGHING YOURSELF AT THE SAME TIME EVERY DAY

To ensure the most progress possible, remember to be consistent in your weighing habits. We giggle each time we remember one lady who was so obsessed with the scale that she weighed herself four, five, and six times a day. Needless to say, this was only stressing her, because the scale would move (up *and* down) all day long. Your weight is affected by the weight of your clothes, what you eat and drink, your activity level, and other factors, all of which can make for substantial fluctuations even in a single day.

To help eliminate some of these variables, make a habit of weighing yourself on the same scale at the same time every day. Your best bet is to weigh yourself first thing in the morning, with no clothes on, after going to the bathroom. Be sure it's before you eat or drink anything and before you get dressed. Even if your scale isn't the most accurate, this consistency will give you a realistic view of your weight-loss progress. In addition, some people opt to weigh daily, while others weigh weekly or monthly so they don't get as frustrated when those plateaus make their presence known. Even if you don't weigh daily, weigh yourself at the same time each time, and under the same circumstances.

or drinking or in your exercise routine. Look at your food journal to review details and identify patterns. Is it time to bump up your protein? Or to cut back on carbs? What about your exercise routine—could it stand a boost or even some small changes? Don't forget to take a look at your water intake as well. Maybe you haven't been getting in that 64-ounce requirement each day. Typically, little changes can kick-start your weight loss again.

A plateau is also a great time to reflect on where you were versus where you are now in your journey. Have you lost a substantial amount of weight? Are you seeing changes and improvements? Are clothes fitting differently? This may be a good time to take some new "after" or "in progress" pictures and compare them to your "before" photos. Take a look at those measurements and see how many inches you have lost overall. That number alone can be pretty staggering. Take out an old belt or old pair of pants that fall off you now. Trying them on ought to bring a smile to your face!

When you think you're stuck and not making any progress, give yourself that wake-up call and let the plateau work its magic. The reminders you give yourself during a plateau can have a big effect and can also refresh your spirit. Look on them as little pockets of time that make you focus on something very important . . . you!

Heading off Head Hunger

After weight-loss surgery, you won't have trouble with physical hunger anymore. If, however, you were in the habit of eating when you were bored, sad, angry, or lonely, you may still have the urge to do that. Or you may feel as though you're not getting enough to eat because you're used to larger portions.

It's likely that everyone—every single one of us—has eaten because of pure emotion at one time or another. Have you ever eaten a cookie just because you knew it was your favorite? Or had a piece of cake because it looked delicious? This is head hunger. Head hunger is eating because your head convinces you it's time to eat, even though your body doesn't need the fuel. True hunger is when your body triggers the senses to let you know it needs fuel. Eating for hunger is about keeping the engine running, which Dan and I call our ding-ding zone. You know when your car's gas tank gets low on fuel and that little sensor in your car goes ding-ding? That's what we equate hunger to.

The pre-op counseling and journaling (to identify dangerous foods and eating patterns) may be enough to get you past this so-called head hunger. If you need more help, therapy will help you find the sources of stress or anxiety that are messing with your head. Signs that you could benefit from further help include:

- Feeling consistently unsatisfied by what you eat
- Never feeling you're losing enough weight
- Finding it impossible to establish new eating habits

Remember that this is stomach surgery and not brain surgery. If you experienced emotional eating issues before surgery, you are still going to have emotional eating issues after surgery. A surgeon can fix your pouch, but he or she can't fix your head or operate on your emotional battles.

Look at your weight-loss journey as a puzzle. Each piece—physical, emotional, psychological—is important and will lead, in the end, to a beautiful and complete picture. How frustrating is it to put together a huge puzzle and discover one or two pieces are missing? It's the same with weight-loss surgery. To create that beautiful result, all the pieces need to fit nicely together. And one of the most important pieces is the psychological side of this procedure—it is, in fact, every bit as important as having a great surgeon. Without your mind in the right place, you're going to constantly battle your food demons.

If you have emotional eating issues and know this is going to be a problem area for you, seek out help. Plenty of eating disorder counselors or bariatric counselors specialize in this exact thing. Don't think of it as shameful—quite the contrary. Kudos to you for wanting to better yourself and giving yourself the best possible chance for success! Whether you choose one-on-one counseling or group sessions, you'll find the minimal investment can change your difficult situation into a manageable one. You might consider looking into this before your surgery, just to give yourself a head start. But even after the surgery, it's never too late to begin if you find yourself struggling with food issues.

Boredom is another factor in head hunger. This isn't just physical boredom but boredom from getting into a food rut or not having your tastes satisfied. A chef will tell you that you eat with your eyes as well as your taste buds, because eating is a very sensory process. You can fill your pouch with anything, but that's just filling the void and not feeding your senses. If you keep your foods interesting and flavorful, you will be more satisfied, and your head will concur with your stomach that it is happy and full.

To prevent head hunger, be sure to eat a variety of foods and flavors after weight-loss surgery. Changing eating habits isn't easy, and learning to cook a new way or with new foods does take some effort. Dan and I make a habit of trying something new each week—a new spice, new herb, or new recipe. It's much easier to stick with recipes we've cooked for years, but for an extra 5 or 10 minutes, we can work in something new. It could result in a new habit and new way of cooking to the point where eventually you don't even think about it. It's also not difficult to take your old favorite recipes and change them up. Spice them up or add another dimension or another flavor layer. Your taste buds, your tummy, and your head will appreciate it.

—————————— **MAKING THE CONNECTION** ——————————

Carolyn's Story: The day after I decided to have gastric bypass surgery, I went to the coffee shop to get my morning fix when a guy slammed the door in my face as I tried to enter. His truck had a bumper sticker that read "No Fat Chicks."

Six months after surgery, 60 pounds lighter, I returned to the shop for my morning decaf. To my surprise, the same man held the door open for me. This time, he smiled as he looked me up and down. He attempted to start a dialogue, but I averted my eyes.

I fight the urge to say, "I am still the same person, why could you not see that?" I feel angry and frustrated at those who judged me by my appearance. I am saddened by the times I was not treated well and wonder how my life might have been different if I hadn't been teased or taunted. If I hadn't been so sad, would I have gotten so big?

But ultimately, I know that it's not only that other people treat me better now; I treat *myself* better now, too. That's the irony of my weight-loss surgery experience.

Expunging Old Habits

Whether it's eating habits or daily routines, we're all creatures of habit. We reach for the same favorites, take the same path, and gravitate to the same places. But now is the time to reevaluate those old habits. Some habits are good ones to keep, but for the most part, bad habits are what got us into trouble in the first place. If you don't change those habits, guess what? You're eventually going to end up right back in the same place.

You didn't have major surgery to let something like bad choices defeat you. I've mentioned journaling throughout this book, and this is one area where cataloging thoughts, foods, portions, and other details about your meals is going to reveal those old habits. Check out the journal pages in Appendix B, and use them to help you change those old habits into new, healthy ones.

You're not an old dog—you *can* learn new tricks. When old habits are converted to new habits, those new habits eventually become old habits. You simply replace the old habits with new, good habits! After a while they aren't new any longer, and you'll be as comfortable in the new as you were with the old.

Repetition is the key to forming new habits. Perhaps you've heard the adage that it takes 21 days to form a habit. Like anything else, there are variables that make this more or less true for certain people. Some people may simply adapt more quickly. Positive or negative reinforcement are also instrumental in making a habit stick. For example, for weight-loss surgery patients, dumping (see Chapter 4) can be a major catalyst in teaching you very quickly not to eat an offending food again. It doesn't mean, however, that everyone learns from this unpleasant experience. If you have dumped only once, you won't be as likely to fear it as if you have dumped 10 times.

One habit we hear a lot regards drinking water. It seems that we all had our favorite "vice" drink before surgery, whether soda, high-caffeine beverage, or high-sugar drink. Before surgery, many people panic about giving up that favorite vice. It turns out, though, that it's usually one of the quickest and easiest habits to reprogram, because the old drink ends up being too filling, causing dumping, or just tasting bad after the surgery.

Keep in mind that although some habits spring from a psychological attachment that can be changed, other habits may have a physical, addictive, or genetic attachment. Some people have food addictions just like some have nicotine, alcohol, or drug addictions and need to seek outside help in working through these addictions and behavior modification. There's also a phenomenon called *transfer addiction*, a psychological transfer in which one's addiction to food is replaced by another obsession, such as shopping or alcohol. It's not a side effect of surgery but a psychological issue. If this sounds like you, find the help you need!

Being Satisfied with Your Successes Along the Way

I can't tell you how many times we hear people say that they have lost "only" 29 pounds in two weeks. Or that they have lost "only" 50 pounds in a month or two. I want to grab them by the shoulders and shake them! When was the last time anyone was able to drop 29 pounds in two weeks? Or 50 pounds in two months? Remember that the weight didn't pack on overnight. To see results of losing a pound or so a day is phenomenal!

Not everyone will lose a pound a day. Some may lose two pounds, while others may lose half a pound a day in those early days. Don't worry about the number! Don't let yourself get so wrapped up in the scale and your end objective that you forget to enjoy the fact that the scale *is indeed* moving, that the inches are dropping, and that you're getting healthier with each passing day. Your losses will be as individual as you are, but the loss numbers and health changes are still mind-boggling.

Get excited about your successes! This is a great time in your life. Fulfill some of your dreams and wishes. Be happy for the person who lost more pounds or lost them faster than you have. Reach out and support another weight-loss surgery patient who may be on a plateau.

If you're a year past your surgery and you have another 20 pounds that's not coming off, you may start to feel that your amazing success is really a failure. Or maybe you wanted to be in a size 4, but your body says you're OK in a 6 or an 8. Don't lose sight of where you started. And remember what's most important: is it a particular number, or is it how you look and feel and having worked your way out of that high-risk health category? With so many improvements in your life and health, don't let a numeric goal—one that may be meaningless in the end—drag you down.

Some people want to be the size they were in high school, but our adult bodies just are not meant to stay child-size. True, a high school student's body isn't small, but it's still not a mature body. One of support group success stories used to weigh over 300 pounds; she is now 150 pounds and a size 6. She described how each major milestone made such a difference in her life, like when she dropped under 300 pounds, then under 200 pounds. But as we talked some more, she mentioned her high school weight, which was 110 pounds. She would be rail thin if she dropped down to that today! But she has an image of her ideal body stuck in her head from many, many years past.

Very rarely is an individual going to regain that teenage body. Why set yourself up for disappointment? Instead, work on and focus on being happy with the new thinner, healthier you. You haven't already forgotten what it was like to struggle with weight, so be proud of yourself and of what you are accomplishing. Be proud of every flaw in your body. No one— not even the very thin—is completely satisfied with his or her body, but you can sure learn to appreciate the difference from your before to your after. It's a transformation that is worth seeing every day. And keep those before and after photos with you as a reminder, too. It's your badge of honor to have gone from that formerly morbidly obese individual to a healthy size for your body type.

Remember, it's *not* about the numbers. It's about your health. It's about how you feel and your quality of life. Love what you've

MAKING THE CONNECTION

Bill's Story: For me, the best change has been my ability to get up and walk since the surgery. I was pretty much crippled by my weight. I used to use a cane to walk—that is, when I could walk. Now, I have a job where I am sometimes on my feet up to eight hours a day! I sometimes still can't believe that I can do that. But I can, and I do! But there are so many little things, too, that I am grateful for as a result of the surgery: I can pick up my kids, and carry them if I want without pain, without my heart feeling like it's going to break out of my chest, without breaking into a sweat, without losing my breath.

I remember the time I was sitting at home watching some TV with my wife. She looked over at me and yelled, "Look what you're doing!" I had no idea what I was doing, so I asked her what. She said "You're crossing your legs!" I hadn't even noticed. I didn't even know I could do that now!

I remember the first time that I realized I could tie my shoes normally. I didn't have to tie them from the side. I didn't have to tie them loosely so that they could be slipped off and on without having to tie them at all.

I recently rode a bike for the first time in over 20 years.

I can go to Disney World and not have to go through the stroller entrance due to my size. I can fit through the turnstile just fine now.

One time, I was shopping for a shirt and the clerk asked me if I needed any help. I said, "Yes, do you have this in a smaller size?"

I no longer fear going to a new restaurant hoping that it would have tables with individual chairs (instead of seats attached to the tables) and that those chairs wouldn't have arms.

I am looking forward to flying. I have a trip scheduled in a couple of weeks, and this will be my first flight since my surgery. I'm not worried about how/if I'll fit into a seat anymore.

It all adds up to an amazing experience. I don't ever want to be that person again, and now with this surgery I feel for the first time that I will never be him again.

accomplished, and love the person you are. You've achieved something to be very proud of.

Seeing Your Body Clearly

Even with the evidence of those photos in front of you, many weight-loss surgery patients find that it takes a whole lot longer for their head to catch up with their body. You may have spent so many years as a morbidly obese individual, berating yourself over your size and shape, that you have fostered many negative feelings about that shape. Now, after losing so much weight, many of us find that even though we know we are much smaller, we still have a hard time seeing that in photos. Many still see that fat person from before. I could look in a mirror and see a smaller person, but I could see a photo and still see that former size 24, not my new size 4. Give yourself time for your brain to catch up with your body. In the end, however, you'll probably need to give yourself permission to *like* the way you look.

The technical term for your brain's inability to see your body clearly is called *body dysmorphic disorder*. With body dysmorphic disorder, no matter how much weight people lose or what they weigh now, they cannot see any positives in their new look. The phrase doesn't apply only to morbidly obese individuals and has many layers of issues and symptoms, some of which we'll discuss in this section. The common thread, though, is the dissatisfaction with the body and the inability to see the positives, instead focusing on real or imagined flaws.

When you're morbidly obese, you may spend hours on end, throughout the weeks, months, and years, criticizing your body. It's no wonder you can't be happy with the results after your surgery and as you lose weight. When you're morbidly obese, you're unhappy with the fat rolls. When you lose weight, you're unhappy because there may be some stretch marks or sagging of the skin. One woman, who lost over 200 pounds, even commented that at least her wrinkles were plumped out when she was fat—but she was unhappy and unhealthy when she was fat.

Be sure you're taking a realistic look at your body and balance what is important. There isn't a one of us who wouldn't love to have that perfect hard body, but what is perfection? Is it the twenty-something who has the high metabolism and works out five hours each day? Is a hard body worth that kind of work? What happens when that individual stops working out? Also, what motivates people to continue to work out like that? When we talked with a group of individuals who fit that description, would you believe that not one of them was satisfied with their bodies? We couldn't see a single flaw, but they each pointed out something they were dissatisfied with. So no matter whether a person is morbidly obese or appears to be our version of perfection, they just are not perfect and never will be. Instead, learn to be happy with who you are, flaws and all. Learn to be happy with what you've accomplished. Learn to love the positives about yourself. It takes more energy to dwell on the negatives than the positives.

If you had your choice of feeling good about yourself or tearing yourself down, which would you prefer? No one wants to feel badly. No one wants to dwell on negatives. This is something you control and you can choose to do. Every time a negative thought pops into your head about a specific body complaint, counter it with a positive. For example:

- My thighs are too big. *Well, they aren't the thighs they were before surgery.*
- My hips are too large. *Well, they must be a lot smaller because I don't have to use a seat extender on a plane any longer.*
- I have some sagging skin. *Sure, but I no longer have fat rolls.*

Remember, there will always be the positives, and they will far outweigh the negatives.

Have you ever seen someone who was morbidly obese, and you thought they were beautiful? Or have you ever seen a thin person who was physically pretty, but you didn't find him or her attractive because of the person's attitude or actions? Size isn't the determining factor in beauty or goodness. That comes from inside, and, believe me, it does come through. If you are happy with yourself, that image will shine through to others and will also be a satisfying quotient in your own life. Reflection isn't just your image in the mirror, it's what you project.

Getting the Support You Need for Life

Do you need support *before* surgery or *after* surgery? In my opinion, both! When you're starting your surgery process, what better place than a support group to get a clear picture of what to expect, especially if members of that group are patients of your surgeon? You can look back to Chapter 4 for more on finding and joining a support group before your surgery.

Receiving support is equally important after surgery. Even though we're long past our own surgery days, Dan and I love opening our e-mails or getting on the message board at thewlsconnection.com to read the enthusiasm of those getting ready for surgery, those who are recent post-ops, and those who are losing rapidly and seeing incredible changes. Not only is their enthusiasm contagious, but it's also a daily reminder that we used to be in that position—at one point, we were just as focused on research or just out of surgery. We remember the excitement of jumping out of bed in the morning to see how far the scale had gone down. We remember the excitement of our clothes getting looser and looser each day.

Even after you reach your maintenance phase, hearing such news from other patients is both exciting and cathartic. You get to cheer the success of others who are following in your footsteps.

But more than that, support groups help you during your maintenance phase in ways you may not be able to imagine. In fact, being connected to a support group is a surefire way to be certain that you never revert to old habits and gain back your old weight. Joining one or more support groups brings an added source of information and comfort for you as the maintenance patient, when you have finally reached your goal and are out of that high-risk health category. There are many places to find ongoing, lifelong support, and this chapter helps you find them.

Understanding the Benefits of Staying Connected

Staying connected plays many parts in long-term weight-loss surgery success. The field of weight-loss surgery is continually changing and growing, as are the products and information for weight-loss surgery patients. By being in that circle of communication, you can stay on top of that information and keep learning from and sharing with other people. It's like having thousands of scouts out there, looking for the best of everything for you—almost like having personal shoppers and cheerleaders rolled into one.

Support isn't just for the good days. You'll probably have days in which you need a swift, yet loving, kick in the pants. It's all about accountability, having people to answer to. We all have vulnerabilities, and no surgery is going to correct that. The key is being aware of and identifying your vulnerabilities in each phase and then using your connection to a support group to keep you living the new, healthy life you've created for yourself.

When you're part of a support group, you'll find that it really is like being part of a family. Each member of the group cares about each other and feels that if even one member fails, everyone fails. The support family cares about and supports you even when you have missteps, helping you get back on track and face the situation. None of us is perfect, but having a support group helps keep you more focused when it comes to your choices and your new habits.

Even after days and years pass, those of us who've had weight-loss surgery live with something that most people will never experience and could never understand. A support community provides a much-needed place of understanding and companionship for the weight-loss surgery patient at any stage of life.

One of our longtime members had weight-loss surgery back in the 1980s, and she's one of the first to tell others in the group how important support is. She's also quick to point out that if she didn't truly believe that, she wouldn't be there herself. She regularly shares her story and her insights. Most important, however, she knows her connection with her support group is what keeps her on the right track.

Have you ever started something and been so excited that you just couldn't get enough of it? Whether it was working out or doing a project or taking a class you always wanted to take, you just couldn't wait until the next opportunity to do it again. After a little while, though, you might skip a gym session or a class. Before you know it, you quit going or doing it. That's simi-

——————————— MAKING THE CONNECTION ———————————

Mary's Story: Now a 15-year weight-loss surgery veteran, I married young and moved with my new husband away from my family so he could attend school. I tried to become a perfect housewife, but I was lonely and unhappy. Within a few months of married life, I noticed my size 12s getting tighter, and my husband began to make little insulting comments. With my feelings hurt, I'd eat. He was making friends at school and work while I was in an apartment with no one but the TV and a kitchen full of food—and food became my friend. When I tried to talk to him about how I felt, he became angry and critical. Soon, I learned to keep my mouth shut and deal the best I could, usually with food.

At age 21, I became pregnant with my daughter. At my first office visit, I stepped on the scale, and it read 240 pounds. Embarrassed by the weight lecture from the doctor, I stopped by Burger King and then cried all the way home. In the two intervening years, my husband graduated from college and got a good-paying job but worked long hours. He didn't want me to go to company functions (I assume it was because he was embarrassed by me), and during that time, my relationship with food grew even stronger. It became my way of dealing with stress and was my best friend. But I was miserable. Then, at 23, I had my son and weighed in at 275 pounds.

I tried every diet known to man. Then, one day, my husband came home from work and told me that a woman at work had gone through gastric bypass surgery and had lost 100 pounds. I was willing to try anything, especially if it meant finally getting love from my husband. I called up the woman for information and then started researching on my own. I saw all that she had lost by being obese, and I wanted to change my life. I started going to a support group in preparation for my surgery.

As it is for so many people, the results of the surgery were amazing, and I lost a total of 218 pounds in 18 months. But it was *after* the surgery that my life really began to change, and that was when I needed support more than ever. Because after all my weight loss, my husband became very jealous. Even with couple's counseling, things went from bad to worse, until my husband, who had always been verbally abusive, became physically abusive. But with support from my group and my therapist, I became my own person and started speaking up for myself. Five years after I'd lost the weight, I left my husband. I loved him so much, but I had learned to love me even more.

---

lar to what can happen with support, if you let it. You get excited about the road ahead and you have this dream of finally reclaiming your life and getting to a healthy weight. Everyone important to you then gives, cares, answers, and supports, gladly and willingly. They walk you through the whats, what ifs, oh nos, oh yesses, and oh mys. They're there for you when you're excited, sad, or scared. They're there for you when you succeed or have a setback. You have your surgery, the weight begins to come off, and you regain that joyous life.

But then life gets busy, and little by little you may forget to go back to your group. It's not that you're turning your back on them. You're just busy now. But one day you get on the scale and see a pound or two come back on. You're not talking to anyone about it and it's just a pound or two, right? While we know it's normal to gain a small amount back (about 10–15 percent of the lost weight), being connected can help you nip that in the bud and drop that pound or two back off before it becomes 20 or 30 pounds. Time and time again, the people who stay connected don't tend to have as many issues down the road.

Support groups talk about it all. From what to expect to emotional upheavals, vitamins, sex, dumping. You name it, it's discussed in a nonthreatening and nonembarrassing environment. As you get involved with a support group, be sure to do the following:

- Learn to feed on the wonderful energy of people who've just had the surgery, sharing in their stories and their accomplishments.
- Share your wisdom with those who are new to the experience.
- Use the opportunity to learn the latest medical advice from others.
- Recognize that your support family can be a truly nurturing family for you, filled with people you'll always be able to rely on.

Finding Support in Your Surgeon's Other Patients

Most surgeons have their own support groups, and bariatric centers typically have regular group meetings. Taking advantage of one of these groups helps you know what to expect from a particular surgeon. Talking with your surgeon's patients also gives you the advantage of making friends *and* seeing success stories before your very eyes.

These support group members can walk you through some of the unknowns. For example, when you go to the hospital, what are the various surgical rooms like? Are family members or friends allowed in with you? Is the staff friendly and reassur-

---
MAKING THE CONNECTION

Gail's Story (Howard's Other Woman): While the success stories are endless, so are the funny little events that can occur with major weight loss. Sometimes, we've gotten so used to seeing our own transformation each day that we forget about other people's reactions.

One day, my husband, Howie, received a phone call at work. This friend calling had received a call from his ex-sister-in-law to tell him she saw Howie with a woman at a restaurant! She was so concerned because she knew us both, and she couldn't believe what she was seeing. What she was seeing was me, though, after losing the equivalent of a large adult's worth of weight! Even after explaining to her, she was still insistent it wasn't Gail because this woman was tiny, and didn't we all know Gail is rather large? She was convinced Howie was stepping out and had a girlfriend, even though he has been a loving and loyal husband for over 30 years. To this day, Howie and I still laugh about his "girlfriend." It's pretty nice to be his trophy wife and his girlfriend without looking like two people rolled into one.

---

ing? Comforting? What was the last thing they remember before waking up in recovery? (Most don't remember getting to the operating room.) There's something very calming about hearing these things from patients at your local facility.

Some people find it intimidating to walk into a face-to-face support group meeting. This may be a throwback to all of those years of feeling invisible or less than worthy purely due to one's size. We've all spent so many years not speaking up or feeling uncomfortable that being very visible can feel foreign. What people forget, though, is that the people in these support groups know *exactly* what that's like, and they are there to encourage you, support you, and guide you.

The first time Dan and I walked into a support group meeting, all these strangers were staring at us, and that felt uncomfortable. We quickly learned, however, that every person there had the same qualms the first time they walked in. In support group, everyone is welcome. Whether listening or participating, everyone is there for a purpose.

When attending a group, take a notepad—you are going to discover a wealth of information and will want to jot down notes. Even if you're a gastric bypass veteran, there's a good chance you'll glean some new information, such as new proteins, vitamins, processes, or recipes, in the meetings.

The biggest disservice you can do to yourself is to not open up. Some people are quite shy and find it hard to make that first comment or ask that first question. But trust me, the people in your group love getting your questions and hearing your stories. And you never know what other shy person you'll inspire by opening up about your own issues! In our local group, we make a point to go around the room. Everyone introduces him- or herself and tells where he or she is in the process, pre- or post-op; how much weight he or she has lost; and more. As each person speaks, something triggers a question or comment, or a success is cheered on by fellow members.

Joys, triumphs, fears, accolades, and accomplishments are all shared in meetings. This is your safe place, a place to voice whatever comes to mind. This is your place to feel comfortable in your own skin, whether you're pre-op or a veteran success story.

Going Online

Online support groups are another incredible resource. Online groups allow you to be just as anonymous or as visible as you

─────────────── MAKING THE CONNECTION ───────────────

Bill and Lee's Story: My husband, Bill, was a diabetic and on insulin for several years. To top it off, he was told by his cardiologist that unless he lost weight, he was surely going to die. Bless his heart, Bill tried every diet he came across and he would lose, like so many, and then gain it all back, with some added padding to boot. My Bill was the perfect Santa: children loved him, and he didn't even have to add padding to his Santa suit. This wasn't a good thing though. We toyed with the idea of gastric bypass but really weren't sure what to do or where to go. He had climbed up to 312 pounds, and along with the heart problems, he also had acquired high blood pressure, COPD [chronic obstructive pulmonary disease], and breathing problems. It was time to do something, and we decided gastric bypass was his last option.

Within one week after surgery, Bill was completely off insulin, and his other medications were cut in half. He has lost his excess weight and has kept it off. The one big drawback now is that *lots* of padding is needed for his Santa suit. We'd say that's a pretty good trade-off. Bill says his biggest gift was finding a surgeon who saved his life and who has now given us a chance to look forward to having a lot of life left to share together.

───

like. People who are particularly shy may find it easier to be a part of a forum in which they don't have to speak up if they don't want to. An online group gives you the chance to see that others have the same questions and to respond after you've had time to think about and consider the questions and comments. You'll also find that while most online support groups have members from all over the world, you have support family as close as a few keystrokes at any time of the day or night.

Are you afraid you might not fit in? That's an easy one: just be yourself. Introduce yourself. Start off by telling who you are or what you would like to be called online (you don't have to use your real name if you don't want to) and saying hello. Elaborate as much as you like. Are you researching or information gathering? Are you in process or looking for a surgeon? Do you have specific questions, concerns, or comments? Nothing makes it easier for individuals in the group to respond than hearing some of your own story. Something as simple as "Hi, my name is . . . and I'm new here" will illicit responses. You're under no pressure to give up information or to answer in any format or time frame. It is courteous, however, to respond in a timely manner.

As with local groups, you get what you give. If you put yourself out there, others will respond and they'll appreciate your responding in kind to them. In short, you will be chatting back and forth with your new support family.

Some guidelines for online groups are pretty simple. Typical online etiquette is usually spelled out in the message board rules. Basic things like being courteous, using appropriate language, no SHOUTING (writing your messages in all caps), no spamming, and no fair being just a taker—that is, someone who takes support and advice but never gives it. Support is a two-way street. Although you don't have to respond to anyone, it would be a pretty sad support group if people only asked questions and never gave answers or feedback or encouragement, don't you think? Remember, no matter how insignificant you may think your comment or question or suggestion is, there's a good chance others have had the same thought or questions, too.

Maintaining Support Even Through Your Maintenance Phase

If you are like most people, for the first 12 to 24 months after surgery you will be really enthusiastic, feel really good, see rapid progress, and be determined to make good choices. Your energy level will be up, you'll get compliments and new surprises every day, and you'll be losing weight faster than you ever dreamed possible. One day, you may even feel you don't need support anymore and walk away from your local or online group. Maybe you've hit your goal and you think: mission accomplished. You're in the maintenance phase—how hard could that be?

Support becomes *more* important after you get to the maintenance level. That's because weight-loss surgery isn't like other surgeries. As I've said before, your stomach was not diseased before your surgery, and your surgeon didn't cure it. You cure yourself by taking the opportunity the surgery provides, but that cure is something you have to maintain every day. When your friends, family, and coworkers are used to the new you, when the dramatic physical changes are over, losing weight can't remain the central focus and main activity of your life. And that's when a lot of people leave their support groups and start to slip. You know how you should be eating, but if there's no feedback from your peers and no accountability to a group, it's easy to lose the focus on healthy food, to stop weighing yourself regularly, and to cut other corners. One morning you may find that you've gained 10 or 20—or even 30 or 40—pounds. Now you start to get concerned. Do you go back to your group, or do you hide the scale?

Stay connected to your support family after you've graduated to the maintenance phase. This connection is as important as the surgery itself. In the early days, you'll find that it's 100 percent the surgery working, with little or no effort on your part. As you progress through the stages those percentages change: 90 percent surgery, 10 percent your efforts; 80 percent surgery, 20 percent you; until it feels as if it's 100 percent you. We know it's not 100 percent you, because the tool is always in place. Over time, however, you can learn to cheat the pouch, which in turn is just cheating yourself. By staying connected to an online support

Tammy's Big Hug: Sometimes it's the small things in a person's weight-loss surgery journey that become the most memorable moments. The best thing that has happened so far since my surgery is that the other day, when my daughter hugged me, she got so excited because she could touch her hands at the back of me. To me, this was a pretty cool moment I will always remember: she said, "Mommy, now I can really hug you!" Need I say more?

---

group during this maintenance phase, you have that accountability factor that is going to be all important in keeping you on track.

Those who have had surgery many years ago have also discovered that the connection is not only a social one but a lifeline with people who understand what their lives are like. This is a major life change, but it is something that most people in your life just aren't going to understand if they haven't experienced it themselves. While others can see the physical changes, they can't be there to answer the questions that may arise along the way. Also, who can appreciate your successes more than your weight-loss surgery peers? Your support family is always there as that lifeline and that anchor to keep you steady, whether it's the first day or 40 years post-op.

Keeping Your Memories Alive

Have you ever had a situation that hurt, such as an injury or a procedure that hurt at the moment? Over time, you forgot the pain and only later did you remember it when you experienced the same thing again. A similar thing can happen with your memories of being morbidly obese or those feelings you had. Don't let them fade.

You learn from your mistakes and experiences. Never take this procedure for granted or slide back into old patterns because you forgot how it felt to carry that extra 100, 200, or 300 pounds around. Don't forget how invisible or miserable you felt. Stay connected to those memories and avoid those pitfalls.

You are who you are because of the paths you've walked so far. Keep those memories fresh and raw. The more you keep those old memories in the forefront of your mind, the more likely you will be to hold your course and stay successful.

Giving Back to the Weight-Loss Surgery Community

When you stay connected, it does more than just feed your psyche. This entire group of individuals can understand where you've been and where you're going. This entire support family has felt the pain and anguish of morbid obesity and has experienced the thrill and victory of losing weight and regaining their lives. There's no other place where you'll find so many who can truly feel your pain or share in your joy.

How good would it feel to give back to this community?

If you have already had the surgery, did you feel all alone when you started the process? Have dozens of questions? When you were packing to go to the hospital, did you feel anxious? When you lost that first 20 pounds, 50 pounds, or 100 pounds were you so excited that you wanted to shout it to the world? Did you turn to your support group? Did they cheer you, cry with you, console, comfort, cajole, and at times even chastise you (in a loving way)? Would you have had the same positive experience without your support group? No way!

——————————— MAKING THE CONNECTION ———————————

Sissy's Story: My heaviest weight was 274 pounds, but in a short two months I've already dropped below 200 pounds! I haven't always been a "big girl," even though I was into sports and very active. When I became pregnant with my first child, like so many others, I gained about 50 pounds. When my first child was two months old, I found out I was pregnant again. I then gained on top of those 50 pounds another 60 pounds.

My kids are now at an age to go to carnivals and ride rides. Every time we would go to Sea World, for example, I would have to make my husband ride with the kids, while I stood by and watched as they had fun. But this year I am going to be able to get on those rides with my kids thanks to gastric bypass surgery. It's the best thing I have ever done for myself, and it's amazing how much I have missed out on because of my weight. But not anymore! I plan to roller coaster myself to dizziness.

Also now I enjoy shopping, and I can now go to "the other side" of the store—you know, where the clothes only go to an XL. It is so wonderful to look at something and think it's too small for me, only to try it on and find that it's a perfect fit. I can't explain the feeling, but it's like your heart is smiling.

Do you remember what a relief it was when you first joined a support group and realized how many understood your feelings? Can you imagine what it would be like to go through this process all alone, with no answers at all? Wondering? Worrying? Guessing? This is why it's important to give back. When interacting with new patients joining your group, keep in mind what it was like for you at their stage of the experience. You get to be like that person at school who shows the new kid around and helps him or her learn everyone's name.

After reading tens of thousands of posts on our message boards, Dan and I still find it energizing. Every day, we get to hear about someone else reaching a new milestone or hitting a goal or getting approved for surgery. Every day, we get to share in the lives of people who would not otherwise have crossed our paths. After so many years of being all but disconnected, we now have a true connection. When I read about someone hitting their first goal or getting the phone call that they are approved for surgery, I get goose bumps. You can hear the enthusiasm and excitement coming through in their posts. In fact, most support group members will tell you that the first thing they think to do when something good happens (approval, goal met, and so on) is to run to the computer and share the news with their online family. That's a connection that goes further than just those keystrokes. That's a true bond, a true connection.

No one should travel this road alone, which makes the benefits of a support group unending. Even after losing weight and walking the right path and enjoying your life, you can still make a difference. Your story and your experiences can mean the difference between someone else succeeding or feeling alone and scared like they have for so many years.

We look at it as the pay-it-forward theory. Others were there for us, and we follow suit and keep paying it forward with a bit of ourselves. Can you even begin to imagine how many people you can truly touch without realizing it? How many lives you can influence for the better? Merely by being a part of the group and sharing a bit of yourself, you help not only yourself but all those who talk with you—and even those who just sit back and listen. What a legacy! After so many years of feeling insignificant or invisible, now you can make a difference—and your support family will continue to make a difference for you as well.

So, remember to remember. Remember the pain. Remember the joys. Remember the past hurts and humiliations. Remember the accomplishments. Remember to stay connected to your support family because that's the place where it's all real for you and where accountability meets your choices and the scale. Remember where you were before surgery, and remember where you are now. Remember that you never want to return to that unhealthy life or lifestyle. Your support connection is your lifeline and your sounding board. Hold onto that connection and treasure it, utilize it, value it. It's for life. For your life. For the rest of your life.

Favorite Recipes

To keep your taste buds happy, here are some of my favorite recipes for you to try. From flavor-filled broths for the weeks following surgery to easy-to-make snacks and dinners, these are all crowd-pleasers and fan favorites!

Just as a side note: Depending on your post-op stage, portion sizes can vary greatly. For a new post-op, a portion may mean two ounces, but a veteran post-op of several years may be able to tolerate six ounces. As I've mentioned time and again, we have to adjust to our own individual body needs. These recipes have serving sizes listed purely for the purpose of determining nutritional information. You make the portions the size that fit your needs.

I hope you enjoy the recipes and will even share recipes of your own. We'd love to hear from you on how you liked these, and we always love adding to our own recipe collection. E-mail us with any comments, recipes you would like to share, suggestions, and more: melissa@connectionwls.com.

Remember, flavor is key to truly being satisfied with your meals. Don't be afraid to experiment and try new things, new recipes, new cooking techniques. Get adventuresome and try new herbs and spices. Something as simple as that can completely change old favorites into new favorites. Enjoy!

Chicken Broth

Makes 20 servings

- 1 whole chicken (2–3 pounds)
- ½-pound package smoked chicken pieces
- 1 large onion, peeled and quartered
- 1 turnip or parsnip, quartered
- 1 head unpeeled garlic, cut in half lengthwise
- 1–2 celery stalks, cut in chunks
- 3 carrots, peeled and cut in half
- 1 bay leaf
- Montreal Steak Seasoning, to taste

Put the whole chicken and the smoked chicken pieces in a stock-pot and cover with about 3 inches of cold water. Simmer for 20 to 30 minutes. Skim off any fatty residue that has accumulated. Add all remaining ingredients and simmer for another 2 to 2½ hours. Discard solids and skim off the broth. Freeze the broth in single-serving containers or ice cube trays.

Note: This same recipe can be converted for a slow cooker. Use the same ingredients, except cut the chicken into pieces. Put all ingredients into a slow cooker and cover with boiling water. Cook on low for 12 hours.

Nutrition information: Per serving: 20 calories, 36% fat (0.2 g; 0g saturated), 0% carbs (0.2 g), 55% protein (4.8 g), 0 g cholesterol, 0 g fiber, 490 mg sodium

Seafood Stock

Makes 20 servings

- 2 pounds seafood or fish (crab, crawfish, and/or shrimp, including shells, or white fish, including bones), rinsed thoroughly
- 1 celery stalk, chopped
- 2 cloves garlic, peeled
- 1 onion, peeled and quartered
- 2 tablespoons chopped parsley

Put all ingredients in a large stockpot and cover with cold water. Simmer for 6 hours. Remove all solids and skim off the broth. Cool and refrigerate or freeze the broth.

Note: You may need to add some water during the simmering process. Make sure the liquid content stays at least 1½ quarts.

Nutrition information: Per serving: 38 calories, 45% fat (1.9 g; 0.5 g saturated), 0% carbs (0 g), 55% protein (5.3 g), 2 g cholesterol, 0 g fiber, 335 mg sodium

Roasted Vegetable Stock

Makes 20 servings

- 1 pound carrots, peeled and quartered
- 3 Vidalia onions, peeled and quartered
- 1 bunch celery, quartered, with leaves removed
- 2 tomatoes, quartered
- 2 red bell peppers, cut in chunks
- 2 orange bell peppers, cut in chunks
- 2 yellow bell peppers, cut in chunks
- 2 sweet potatoes, peeled and quartered
- 2 turnips, quartered
- 2–3 tablespoons olive oil
- 2 cloves of garlic, whole
- 1 bay leaf
- Montreal Steak Seasoning, to taste

Preheat oven to 450°F. Toss vegetables with the olive oil and place in roasting pan. Roast for approximately 1 hour or until vegetables are nicely browned. Transfer ingredients to stockpot and add garlic, bay leaf, and Montreal Steak Seasoning. Cover with water and bring to a boil. Reduce heat and simmer approximately 2 to 3 hours. Strain vegetables. Chill. Pour into individual containers and refrigerate or freeze.

Note: You can also use fresh, seasonal vegetables to replace the veggies listed in the ingredients.

Nutrition information: Per serving: 63 calories, 31% fat (2.3 g; 0.3 g saturated), 63% carbs (6.8 g), 5% protein (1.3 g), 0 g cholesterol, 0 g fiber, 401 mg sodium

Meat Stock

Makes 20 servings

- 2 tablespoons olive oil
- 3–4 pounds any meat and bones, cut into chunks (may be smoked for additional flavor)
- 1 large onion, quartered
- 2–3 celery stalks, chopped
- 2–3 carrots, peeled and halved
- 1 garlic head, cut in half
- 1 bay leaf
- Montreal Steak Seasoning, to taste

Place the olive oil in the stockpot and heat. Add the meat and bone pieces. Cook until browned on all sides, scraping up all the bits on the bottom of the pan as you go. Add the remaining ingredients and cover with water. Bring to a boil. Reduce heat and simmer approximately 2½ to 3 hours, until the meat is tender. Discard meat, bones, and vegetables. Skim off the broth and refrigerate. Once chilled, skim fat from the top, and then freeze into individual portions.

Nutrition information: Per serving: 31 calories, 6% fat (0.2 g; .1 g saturated), 37% carbs (2.8 g), 61% protein (4.7 g), 0 g cholesterol, 0 g fiber, 473 mg sodium

Parmesan Crisps

Makes 8 servings

This is a great high-protein, crispy treat.

- 1 cup freshly grated Parmesan
- Fresh ground pepper, optional

Preheat oven to 400°F. Place a spoonful of parmesan on non-stick baking sheet and press down to form a circle. Repeat, spacing 1 inch apart. Bake for 5 minutes or until melted and crisp. Let cool. Carefully, without breaking, remove crisps from baking sheet.

Nutrition information: Per serving: 54 calories, 58% fat (3.6 g; 2.2 g saturated), 4% carbs (0.5 g), 38% protein (4.8 g), 11 g cholesterol, 0 g fiber, 191 mg sodium

Roll-ups

These are easy, high-protein snacks. Mix it up and get creative. The following are a few of our favorites.

Just layer items and roll up for a quick snack:

- Ham, Jarlesberg, deli mustard
- Smoked turkey, fontina
- Smoked chicken, bacon, Gouda
- Smoked salmon, cream cheese, chopped boiled egg, dollop of sour cream, capers
- Roast beef, fontina, horseradish sauce (horseradish and sour cream)
- Ham, scrambled egg, cheese (good for breakfast)
- Prosciutto, mozzarella, thin slice of cantaloupe
- Turkey, pepper jack cheese, slice or two of avocado
- Chicken, mozzarella, thin layer of marinara sauce (just enough for flavor)
- Ham, turkey, or chicken, cream cheese, asparagus spear for crunch
- Smoked turkey, radish sprouts, cheese of your choice, sunflower seeds
- Lettuce leaf, bacon, cheese, dab of mayonnaise
- Lettuce leaf, shrimp, avocado or asparagus, cream cheese

Check deli nutrition information for the specific ingredients in your roll-up creation.

Quick and Easy Cheesy Ham Breakfast Bake

Makes 1 serving

- 3 thin slices deli ham (or other deli meat of your choosing)
- 1–2 slices of your favorite cheese, quartered
- 1 tablespoon chopped green chiles
- 1 egg
- Optional garnish: crushed pork rinds or a few potato sticks for crunch

Preheat oven to 375°F. In a ramekin (or muffin pan), line ham slices to the shape of the baking dish. Place ¾ of cheese over ham and top with green chiles. Cover chiles with remaining cheese. Crack egg over top. Bake for about 17 minutes or until egg reaches desired doneness.

Note: The green chiles are what set this dish apart. Even company loves this one at our house!

Nutrition information: Per serving: 375 calories, 61% fat (25.5 g; 12.7 g saturated), 5% carbs (4 g), 34% protein (30 g), 278 g cholesterol, 1.3 g fiber, 1,632 mg sodium

Garlic Shrimp

Makes 4 servings

- 3 tablespoons extra virgin olive oil
- 3–4 cloves garlic, minced
- ½ pound shrimp, shelled and deveined
- ¼–½ teaspoon crushed red pepper, to taste
- Salt, to taste (sea salt is a great flavor here)

Heat oil in a heavy skillet (use cast iron for added flavor).

Add garlic and cook until it begins to turn a golden color. Add shrimp and cook, stirring, about 2 to 3 minutes. Stir in the rest of the ingredients and immediately remove from heat.

Variations: Alternate or add ingredients such as Spanish paprika, coriander, bay leaf, asparagus, squeeze of lemon, or flat-leaf (Italian) parsley. Freshly grated cheese adds another flavor dimension and additional protein.

Nutrition information: Per serving: 153 calories, 64% fat (11 g; 1.6 g saturated), 3% carbs (1.3 g), 32% protein (12 g), 86 g cholesterol, 0.1 g fiber, 85 mg sodium

Ham, Cheese, and Spanish Chorizo Stacks

Makes 4 servings

While this is a simple recipe, it has great flavor and is loaded with protein.

- 2–3 tablespoons extra virgin olive oil
- ½ pound Spanish chorizo (no substitution), sliced thick
- ¼ pound Serrano ham
- 2 ounces Monterey Jack, sliced

Heat olive oil in skillet. Sauté the chorizo for about 5 minutes. Remove from pan and drain on paper towel. Make stacks: a slice of ham, then a slice of cheese, then a piece of chorizo on top.

Variation: Use different cheeses, such as cheddar or mozzarella.

Nutrition information: Per serving: 317 calories, 73% fat (26 g; 11.8 g saturated), 2% carbs (1.1 g), 25% protein (19 g), 72 g cholesterol, 0 g fiber, 876 mg sodium

Garlic Meatballs

Makes 4 servings

- 1 pound lean ground beef or ground chuck
- ½ small Vidalia onion, chopped
- 2 cloves garlic, minced
- 1 teaspoon Worcestershire sauce
- 1 egg
- ¼ cup evaporated milk or whole milk
- ¼ cup dried bread crumbs (plain or Italian)
- Salt and pepper, to taste
- 1–2 tablespoons vegetable oil

Combine all ingredients except vegetable oil and shape into meatballs. Heat oil in a large skillet and cook meatballs, covered, approximately 15 to 20 minutes. Serve immediately.

Note: Depending on how lean your ground beef is, you may opt to not use the oil for cooking the meatballs. These also freeze well.

Variation: For a Moroccan variation, add 2 tablespoons chopped flat-leaf parsley, 1 tablespoon cumin, ½ teaspoon ground ginger, and ½ tablespoon Tex-Mex seasoning. Top with sauce:

SAUCE

- 1 can tomato sauce
- 1 15-ounce can whole or crushed tomatoes
- ½ teaspoon Tex-Mex seasoning
- 1 clove garlic, minced
- Optional: top with shredded cheese of your choice

Combine all ingredients, pour over meatballs, and simmer until meatballs reach desired doneness. This is a great option for a slow cooker as well.

Nutrition information: Per serving: 607 calories, 73% fat (49.2 g; 19.8 g saturated), 8% carbs (11.2 g), 19% protein (27.6 g), 173 g cholesterol, 1.5 g fiber, 597 mg sodium

---

Shrimp and Scallop Salsa Style

Makes 6 servings

- ½ pound scallops
- ½ pound cooked shrimp, peeled and deveined
- 2–3 tablespoons extra virgin olive oil
- 2 cups salsa (jarred or fresh)
- 1 tomato, diced
- 3 tablespoons chopped cilantro
- Juice of ½ lime
- Salt, to taste

Sauté scallops and shrimp in olive oil. Chill until cool. Dice seafood into bite-sized pieces. Combine remaining ingredients. Stir in shrimp and scallops. Chill.

Note: Precooked or frozen shrimp are a fast alternative for a quick and tasty preparation.

Variations: Chopped avocado adds a nice flavor and texture to this recipe. Use Rotel Tomatoes & Green Chiles in place of the salsa. Experiment with various shellfish, such as lobster or crawfish, and try different varieties of shrimp.

Nutrition information: Per serving: 142 calories, 35% fat (5.6 g; 0.8 g saturated), 20% carbs (7.8 g), 45% protein (15.5 g), 70 g cholesterol, 1.7 g fiber, 637 mg sodium

Chicken and Red Peppers

Makes 4 servings

- ½ cup mayonnaise
- 1 small red bell pepper, chopped fine
- ½ teaspoon crushed red pepper
- 1–2 cloves garlic, minced
- ½ pound boneless, skinless chicken, cut into ½-inch pieces
- 6 wooden skewers (soaked in water)

Combine first four ingredients to create marinade. Place chicken pieces onto wooden skewers and place in shallow dish. Pour marinade over skewers. Cover with plastic wrap and refrigerate for 1 to 3 hours.

Remove skewers and discard any remaining marinade. Place skewers on heated grill or under broiler. Cook for 8 to 10 minutes, turning as needed to obtain desired doneness. Serve immediately.

Variations: This recipe works well with fish (tuna, tilapia, grouper, and more) as well as poultry. Try a variety of peppers, such as orange or yellow bell peppers or sweet roasted peppers. Replace crushed red pepper with a variety of fresh peppers, such as minced serranos or jalapenos, for a different flavor.

Nutrition information: Per serving: 194 calories, 30% fat (6.5 g; 1.1 g saturated), 10% carbs (4 g), 61% protein (27.7 g), 72 g cholesterol, 0.5 g fiber, 182 mg sodium

Citrus and Spice Marinated Skirt Steak

Makes 2 servings

- 1 tablespoon orange juice or pineapple juice concentrate (thawed)
- 1 teaspoon paprika or crushed red pepper
- Salt, to taste
- 1 garlic clove, minced
- 1 teaspoon extra virgin olive oil
- ½ pound skirt steak, trimmed
- Roasted red peppers
- Goat cheese

Combine juice concentrate, paprika or red pepper, salt, garlic, and olive oil. Rub mixture onto steak, covering all sides. Place in a tightly covered container or zip storage bag and refrigerate for 1 to 2 hours.

Grill or sauté steak 2 to 3 minutes on each side or to desired doneness. Let meat rest for approximately 10 minutes so you don't lose the juices when slicing. Slice steak thinly, on a diagonal. Layer steak, roasted red peppers, and goat cheese. Roll and slice.

Variations: Thinly slice fresh, seasonal vegetables, such as asparagus, tomatoes, yellow squash, zucchini, cucumbers, or red onion, and layer with the skirt steak. Experiment with different cheeses, such as bleu, fontina, mozzarella, Gouda, or Gruyère.

Nutrition information: Per serving: 281 calories, 59% fat (18.8 g; 10.3 g saturated), 4% carbs (3.3 g), 37% protein (25 g), 70 g cholesterol, 0.8 g fiber, 140 mg sodium

Spaghetti Squash Cheese Bake

Makes 4 servings

- 1 small spaghetti squash
- 6–8 slices bacon or ½ cup chopped ham or prosciutto
- 8 ounces grated cheddar cheese
- Salt and pepper, to taste

Preheat oven to 350°F. Cut squash in half lengthwise and scoop out and discard seeds.In a small baking dish, place squash skin side up and add ½ to 1 inch of water to pan. Bake for 35 to 40 minutes, until squash is tender. Let cool.

While squash is baking, fry bacon until crisp. Drain. Crumble and set aside.

After the squash has cooled, take a fork and pull the squash out of its skin. This will produce strands similar to spaghetti.

In a medium-sized bowl, combine squash strands, bacon crumbles, grated cheddar cheese, salt, and pepper. Mix until thoroughly coated.

Place mixture back into baking dish. Bake for 5 to 10 minutes at 350°F. If desired, more cheese may be sprinkled on the top. Serve immediately.

Nutrition information: Per serving: 354 calories, 80% fat (31.6 g; 13.8 g saturated), 6% carbs (5.7 g), 16% protein (14 g), 66 g cholesterol, 0 g fiber, 590 mg sodium

Mini Cheesy Bacon Meatloaf

Makes 4 servings

- 2 eggs
- 12 club crackers, crushed
- 1 tablespoon Worcestershire sauce
- ¼ cup chopped onion
- 1 clove garlic, minced
- ½ cup grated cheddar cheese (reserve small amount to sprinkle on top of loaves)
- ½ teaspoon sea salt
- ½ teaspoon ground pepper
- 1 pound ground chuck or lean ground beef
- 4 slices bread (any kind)
- 4 slices bacon

Preheat oven to 350°F. In large bowl combine eggs, crackers, Worcestershire, onion, garlic, cheese, salt, and pepper. Mix in ground chuck. Divide and form into four small loaves. Place the four slices of bread on an ungreased baking sheet (to absorb grease from the meatloaf), and top each slice with one meatloaf. Cut bacon in half and place two pieces on top of each meatloaf.

Bake for 40 minutes. Top with extra cheese and heat until melted. Remove from oven and let rest. Discard bread. Serve hot.

Nutrition information: Per serving: 542 calories, 56% fat (34 g; 13 g saturated), 14% carbs (18.2 g), 30% protein (38.8 g), 235 g cholesterol, 0.7 g fiber, 746 mg sodium

Slow Cooker Tex-Mex Chicken

Makes 8 servings

- 4 boneless, skinless chicken breasts
- 1 package taco seasoning or fajita seasoning
- 1 cup salsa
- 1 can cream of mushroom soup
- ½ cup sour cream

Place chicken in bottom of slow cooker. Sprinkle seasoning mix over top. Layer on salsa and add cream of mushroom soup. Cook on low heat for 6 to 8 hours. Stir in sour cream and serve.

Nutrition information: Per serving: 175.3 calories, 20% fat (3.9 g; 1.7 g saturated), 11% carbs (5.3 g), 69% protein (28.6 g), 75 g cholesterol, 0.7 g fiber, 397 mg sodium

Crab and Avocado Salad

Makes 4 servings

- 2 teaspoons mayonnaise
- 2 teaspoons lime juice
- ¼ teaspoon paprika
- ½ teaspoon cumin
- ½ pound lump crab meat (cooked)
- ¼ cup grated celery root or 1 celery stalk, diced
- 1 ripe avocado, peeled and cubed
- Salt and pepper, to taste

Mix mayonnaise, lime juice, paprika, and cumin. Stir in crab and celery root, being careful not to break up the crab too much. Stir in avocado, taking care not to overmix. Serve immediately.

Nutrition information: Per serving: 148 calories, 48% fat (8.3 g; 1.1 g saturated), 12% carbs (4.8 g), 41% protein (14.4 g), 41 g cholesterol, 3.1 g fiber, 403 mg sodium

Asian Grilled Tuna

Makes 2 servings

- 2 tablespoons orange juice
- 1 tablespoon sesame oil
- 1 teaspoon black or white sesame seeds
- 2 tablespoons light soy sauce
- 2 teaspoons freshly grated ginger (2 teaspoons ground ginger can be substituted)
- ½ pound sashimi-grade tuna

In a plastic bag, mix orange juice, sesame oil, sesame seeds, soy sauce, and ginger. Add tuna and seal. Coat all sides. Marinate for 20 to 30 minutes.

Grill or broil tuna for 2 to 4 minutes per side. With good-quality tuna, rare is preferred.

Note: Pan searing works on this as well. In a hot sauté pan, add a light spray of olive oil. Cook tuna 2 to 3 minutes on each side.

Nutrition information: Per serving: 227 calories, 39% fat (10.2 g; 1.6 g saturated), 8% carbs (4.6 g), 53% protein (28.4 g), 51 g cholesterol, 0.7 g fiber, 210 mg sodium

Oven-Roasted Ranch Chicken

Makes 8 servings

- 1 package (4 ounces) dry buttermilk ranch salad dressing mix
- ⅓ cup plain bread crumbs
- 4 boneless, skinless chicken breasts, halved
- ⅓ cup sour cream
- Cooking spray

Preheat oven to 375°F. On a plate or in a shallow dish, mix ranch dressing mix and bread crumbs. Dip chicken in sour cream and then roll in dressing mixture. Coat well. Place chicken on a non-stick baking sheet, and coat with cooking spray.

Bake for 30 minutes or until chicken is tender and juices run clear.

Nutrition information: Per serving: 169 calories, 20% fat (3.7 g; 1.7 g saturated), 9% carbs (3.6 g), 71% protein (28.1 g), 73 g cholesterol, 0.2 g fiber, 117 mg sodium

Journal Pages: Your Weight-Loss Surgery Connection

Top 10 Wish List

What things do you envision doing? Do you have a list of health issues to be rid of? Things you want to do, places to go, or things to experience? These are your dreams for you.

1. _____
_____

2. _____
_____

3. _____
_____

4. _____
_____

5. _____
_____

6. _____
_____

7. _____
_____

8. _____
_____

9. _____
_____

10. _____
_____

Dreams and Wishes

Fears

Do you have fears about obesity? Surgery? The potential of failure? The unknown? Write down your fears, and then spend time researching what you need to know to alleviate those fears. Talk with your surgeon or bariatric counselor or look to your support group. Don't let your fears sit there. Address them head-on.

Why You Will Succeed with This Surgery

The mind is quite powerful. It's just as easy to succeed as it is to fail, but success feels so much better. Write down why you *will* succeed. This list will grow and change regularly. Review it daily as a reminder. Include the small successes and the large ones. It could be success at developing a new habit (drinking water instead of sodas, taking your vitamins, etc.), or it could be determination and a positive outlook. You decide what makes your success story.

_____

_____

_____

_____

_____

_____

_____

_____

_____

_____

_____

_____

_____

_____

_____

_____

_____

_____

Items to Buy for After the Surgery

As you discover things that will be beneficial after surgery, make a list so you can stock up beforehand. This could include vitamins, supplements, bottled water varieties, books, recipes, or other items.

_____

_____

_____

_____

_____

_____

_____

_____

_____

_____

_____

_____

_____

_____

_____

_____

_____

_____

_____

_____

_____

_____

_____

_____

_____

Items to Pack for the Hospital

Keep it light and remember to leave valuables at home. Keep in mind that you want to be comfortable (see Chapter 4 for ideas). It's the simple things that usually mean the most when you get to the hospital.

Presurgery Measurements

Date: _____

Neck: _____

Chest: _____

Bust: _____

Waist: _____

Hips: _____

Abdomen: _____

Thighs: (right) _____ (left) _____

Calves: (right) _____ (left) _____

Ankles: (right) _____ (left) _____

Upper arms: (right) _____ (left) _____

Lower arms: (right) _____ (left) _____

Wrists: (right) _____ (left) _____

Thoughts About Getting Ready for Surgery

Are you excited? Wondering what it'll be like? Jot down your thoughts, anxieties, excitement, and more. Use this as a tool to discuss these things with your support group as well to answer your questions.

_____

_____

_____

_____

_____

_____

_____

_____

_____

_____

_____

_____

_____

_____

_____

_____

_____

_____

_____

_____

_____

_____

_____

_____

_____

_____

_____

_____

Questions for the Surgeon

As you research and go through the testing and learning process, keep a list of questions for your surgeon. Don't rely on memory, and don't think any question is too small. If it's important enough for you to wonder about, it's important enough to ask.

_____

_____

_____

_____

_____

_____

_____

_____

_____

_____

_____

_____

_____

_____

_____

_____

_____

_____

_____

_____

_____

_____

_____

_____

_____

_____

_____

Goals

Do you have dreams of how your life will change after surgery? Maybe you want to find a new career or go back to school. Maybe it's walking the neighborhood or running a marathon. Your possibilities are endless.

Before Surgery: My Story

Write your journey—the highs and lows and what led you to this point. This is where you're putting that old you in the past. Free yourself up for the road ahead.

_____

_____

_____

_____

_____

_____

_____

_____

_____

_____

_____

_____

_____

_____

_____

_____

_____

_____

_____

_____

_____

_____

_____

_____

_____

_____

Food Journal

Use this section to really pay attention to all aspects of your eating and your choices. Weigh or measure your portions and note them. Don't forget to keep track of the nutrition information: check the protein, carbohydrates, sugars, and more. Describe what you're eating, when, why, how fast, how it tastes, what the texture is like, and even how you feel after you eat it. This exercise will help you develop the habit of paying attention to your food and how it affects you. Do you feel more energetic? Tired? Hungry soon after? All are clues for you.

Favorite restaurants

_____
_____
_____
_____
_____
_____
_____
_____
_____
_____
_____
_____
_____
_____

The names of particularly helpful staff

_____
_____
_____
_____
_____
_____
_____
_____
_____
_____
_____
_____
_____
_____

Restaurant items or specialties

Memorable dining-out or party experiences

My Journey

This is for anything you want to write about—whether it's the events of the day or your feelings, a goal you've reached or a new size. It's all about you and the changes you'll see each day.

Favorite Recipes

If you find something that works particularly well for you, jot it down. Or better yet, develop your own by modifying some of your existing favorites.

Schedule of Appointments

Jot down your list of appointments, schedules, tests, labs, and more.

My First . . .

Your first goal reached, your first hundred pounds lost, your first time to hit a certain weight—there will be lots of firsts, so list them all and relive them frequently.

_____

_____

_____

_____

_____

_____

_____

_____

_____

_____

_____

_____

_____

_____

_____

_____

_____

_____

_____

_____

_____

_____

_____

_____

_____

_____

_____

_____

_____

Converting to Metrics

Volume Measurement Conversions

U.S.	Metric
¼ teaspoon	1.25 ml
½ teaspoon	2.50 ml
¾ teaspoon	3.75 ml
1 teaspoon	5.00 ml
1 tablespoon	15.00 ml
¼ cup	62.50 ml
½ cup	125.00 ml
¾ cup	187.50 ml
1 cup	250.00 ml

Weight Measurement Conversions

U.S.	Metric
1 ounce	28.4 g
8 ounces	227.5 g
16 ounces (1 pound)	455.0 g

Cooking Temperature Conversions

Celsius/Centigrade: 0°C and 100°C are arbitrarily placed at the melting and boiling points of water and standard to the metric system.

Fahrenheit: Fahrenheit established 0°F as the stabilized temperature when equal amounts of ice, water, and salt are mixed.

To convert temperatures in Fahrenheit to Celsius, use this formula:

$$C = (F - 32) \times 0.5555$$

So, for example, if you are baking at 350°F and want to know that temperature in Celsius, use this calculation:

$$C = (350 - 32) \times 0.5555 = 176.65°C$$

References

American Society for Metabolic & Bariatric Surgery, "Rationale for Treatment of Morbid Obesity," asbs.org/Newsite07/patients/resources/asbs_rationale.htm.

Bariatric Edge, "Learn About the Procedures," bariatricedge.com/dtcf/pages/3_Procedures.htm.

Fussy, Sarah A., "The Skinny on Gastric Bypass," *U.S. Pharmacist*, uspharmacist.com/index.asp?show=article&page=8_1438.htm.

New York Times, "Surgical Treatment for Diabetes," January 24, 2008, nytimes.com/2008/01/24/opinion/24thu2.htm.

United States National Library of Medicine, "How to Determine Your BMI," nlm.nih.gov/medlineplus/ency/article/007196.htm.

Index

About the Author

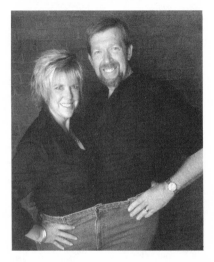

MELISSA DEBIN-PARISH and her husband, Dan, underwent weight-loss surgery in 2003. Melissa has gone from a size 24 down to a size 4, losing 120 pounds, and Dan has gone from a size 54 to a size 32, losing 180 pounds. As a leader of a bariatric surgery support group, Ms. deBin-Parish offers patients great enthusiasm and willingness to share her experiences with this life-changing procedure. She hosts an online website and message board and works with more than ten thousand patients monthly in dealing with the emotional, physical, and social aspects of obesity and morbid obesity.

Today, Melissa and Dan have become two of the country's most sought-after lay experts on weight-loss surgery. Melissa has been recognized as a "bariatric expert on support" by BariMD, a "comprehensive web destination" for bariatric professionals, and she has been elected to the advisory board for the Obesity Action Coalition (obesityaction.org), a national advocacy group. Melissa and Dan speak at events around the country and are frequently invited to help set up new weight-loss support groups in the cities they visit.

Come join her at: thewlsconnection.com, connectionwls .com, http://connectionwls.mywowbb.com, http://groups.msn .com/gastricbypasssupport